NATURAL
REMEDIES
FOR
HAYFEVER

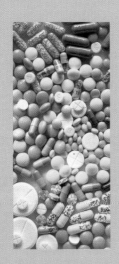

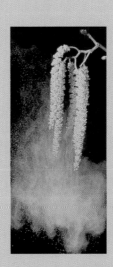

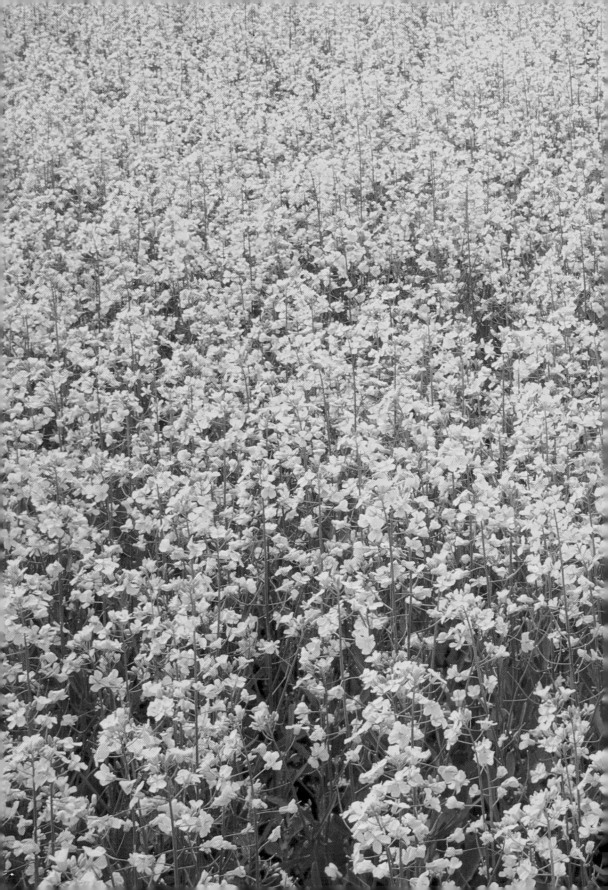

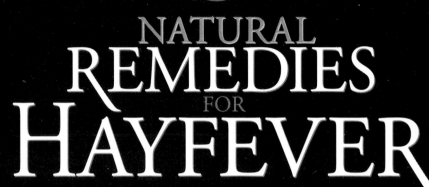

NATURAL
REMEDIES
FOR
HAYFEVER

SELF-HELP MEASURES FOR
TREATING THE SYMPTOMS
OF HAYFEVER NATURALLY

PAUL MORGAN

First published in Great Britain in 1998 by
Parragon
13 Whiteladies Road
Clifton
Bristol BS11 9QD

ISBN: 0-75252-536-0

Produced by Haldane Mason, London

Acknowledgements
Art Director: Ron Samuels
Editorial Director: Sydney Francis
Editorial Consultant: Christopher Fagg
Project Editor: Jo-Anne Cox
Designer: Zoë Mellors
Illustrator: Stephen Dew
Picture Research: Jo-Anne Cox

Printed in Spain

Picture acknowledgements
Dyson: 106; **The Garden Picture Library:** Brian Carter 16, John Glover 17 (bottom), Vaughan Fleming 18, Brian Carter 96, John Glover 112, JS Sira (top), Densey Clyne (bottom) 113; **Haldane Mason:** 6, 21 (top right), 42 (bottom left, top right), 54 (bottom left, top left), 57, 107; **The Healthy House:** 105, 108; **Parragon:** 40 (both), 41 (bottom right), 42 (centre left, centre right), 47, 48, 50, 51 (bottom left), 52, 53, 54 (top right, centre left x 2, centre right), 55 (bottom left, bottom right), 63, 90; **The Royal College of Physicians:** 7; **The Science Photo Library:** Rosenfeld Images Ltd (bottom left), Paul Biddle & Tim Malyon (bottom centre), Dr Jeremy Burgess (bottom right) 1, Kaj R. Svensson 2-3, Rosenfeld Images Ltd (top), Paul Biddle & Tim Malyon (centre), Dr Jeremy Burgess (bottom) 5, John Durham 8, Damien Lovegrove 9, Rosenfeld Images Ltd 10, Damien Lovegrove 11, Biophoto Associates 13, Secchi-Lecaque/Roussel-UCLAF/CNRI (bottom left, bottom centre), Damien Lovegrove (centre, bottom right) 15, Phil Jude 17 (top), Eye of Science 19, Damien Lovegrove 21 (bottom), Mark Clarke 23, Eye of Science 25, Larry Mulvehill 27, John Bavosi 28, Sheila Terry 33, Simon Fraser 35, Rosenfeld Images Ltd 37, Paul Biddle & Tim Malyon 38, Tony Craddock 41 (main), Sheila Terry 43, Ed Young/Agstock 45, Hattie Young 46, Hattie Young 49, Paul Biddle 51 (top), Erika Craddock 55 (top), Damien Lovegrove 62, Damien Lovegrove 65, Paul Biddle & Tim Malyon 66, Damien Lovegrove 75, Peter Menzel 85, Oscar Burriel 86, Alexander Tsiaras 89, Dr Jeremy Burgess 92, Somatino, Jerrican 93, James King-Holmes 98, SIU 99, Dr Vic Bradbury 101, Somatino, Jerrican 110, James King-Holmes 111;.**The Society of Teachers of the Alexander Technique:** 83.

IMPORTANT

The information, recipes and remedies contained in this book are generally applicable and appropriate in most cases, but are not tailored to specific circumstances or individuals. The author and publishers cannot be held responsible for any problems arising from the mistaken identity of any plants or remedies, or the inappropriate use of any remedy or recipe. Do not undertake any form of self diagnosis or treatment for serious complaints without first seeking medical advice. Always seek professional medical advice if symptoms persist.

Contents

Introduction

The history of hayfever

It seems strange to talk about the 'history' of a medical condition, but the fact is that hayfever – or allergic rhinitis, as doctors sometimes call it – is a fairly modern condition. In 1565 one Leonardo Botallo gave the name 'rose cold' to the catarrh and asthma that a few people suffered near blooming roses, but it was not until 1819 that hayfever was identified. Then London doctor John Bostock christened the seasonal nose irritation from which he suffered 'Bostock's summer catarrh'.

Various scientists worked out that pollen was responsible for causing hayfever during the 1870s, and then Wilhelm Dunbar, a German researcher, proved that the condition was the result of an allergy to pollen – though the word 'allergy' was not to be coined for another ten years. Nevertheless, hayfever was now firmly on the medical map, and work continued throughout the century to identify its precise mechanisms. However, it was not until the mid-1970s that scientists were finally able to unlock the puzzle and explain exactly how an allergen works, in terms of what substance is released by which cells in response to the presence of a foreign body to which there is an allergy.

SUMMER CATARRH

While the scientists pondered and experimented, however, the general public was becoming increasingly more aware of hayfever. When Bostock had originally named his 'summer catarrh' in 1819, the condition had been extremely rare: he commented that it had not 'been noticed as a specific affection until within the last ten or twelve years.' At the time, it seemed to be confined exclusively to the very well-to-do, though by the 1870s it had spread to the middle classes – Dr Charles Blackley, who specialised in researching and treating hayfever, noted that it seemed only to affect educated and professional people; indeed, having an attack of hayfever was something of a status symbol.

ONE TEENAGER IN SIX

Hayfever was not to maintain this exclusivity, however, for by the early 1900s, it was a common complaint, and the theory was that it was due to a sensitivity to a new variety of straw – which is why it came to be known as 'hayfever'. In fact, by the 1920s hayfever had become so common that Noel Coward even titled one of his new plays *Hay Fever*. And, remarkably, the number of those who suffer from the condition has continued to rise, to the point that today one in six teenagers is affected. Why? Nobody knows, although there are plenty of theories – all of them, however, remain unproved.

THE ALTERNATIVE PATH

This general sense of uncertainty is not just confined to questions about the incidence of hayfever, but to its medical treatment as well. In the short term, pills and potions can help to relieve symptoms:

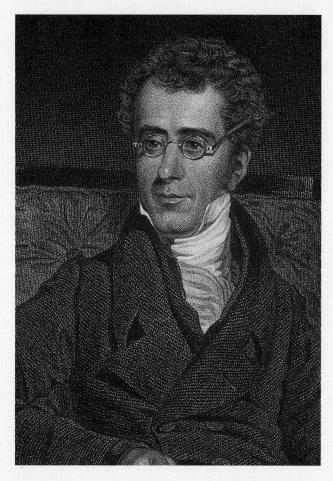

Dr John Bostock, the London doctor who identified hayfever, and named it 'Bostock's catarrh' in 1819.

modern medicine's chemical arsenal of antihistamines, corticosteroids, sympathomimetics and mast cell stabilisers all have their uses – but there is a risk of side-effects of one degree or another with all of them. As far as the long-term results are concerned, the only answers that conventional medicine has to hayfever are time-consuming, costly and not effective in every case.

As a result of these disadvantages, more and more people are turning to an alternative, natural approach to the treatment and prevention of hayfever. They are looking to alternative remedies: to more natural ways of treating an attack of hayfever and reducing the risk that one will develop by means of a combination of holistic therapies and more down-to-earth preventive measures. And the purpose of this book is to give people the information to do just that.

Profile of a hayfever sufferer

If you've bought this book, you are probably one of the millions of people around the world who suffer from hayfever or allergic rhinitis (there are a variety of substances, other than pollen, which cause the same allergic response). That means that you probably have something in common with most hayfever sufferers, but not nearly as much as you might think.

We will look at the genetic basis of hayfever later in the book (see pages 30-31), but it is likely that other members of your family are affected by it or by other allergies to one degree or other, and it is probable that you first experienced the symptoms of hayfever in your teenage years or early twenties – though on rare occasions people develop hayfever in their thirties or forties. You may well have had eczema when you were a child – between 40 and 60 per cent of those who do develop hayfever or asthma later in life.

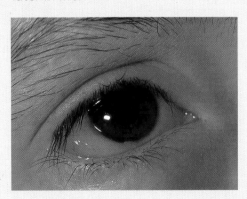

Extraordinarily, you are also likely to be an only child or one of the eldest children in your family. Research has shown that if you are the youngest of five children your chances of developing hayfever are 75 per cent less than if you are the eldest child.

Unfortunately, that's really all that be said about you. We can't deduce, for example, anything about where you work or live, even though many people think that environmental factors, such as pollution, play some part in causing hayfever – but there's really no firm evidence to support this idea. It's true that polluted air or the exhaust fumes you might breathe in a busy town can make an attack of hayfever worse, but they don't trigger the condition. Therefore, it would be pure speculation to make

Hayfever affects the eyes just as much as the nose, causing watering, inflammation and itchiness. Sometimes, the eyes show the only symptoms of a hayfever attack.

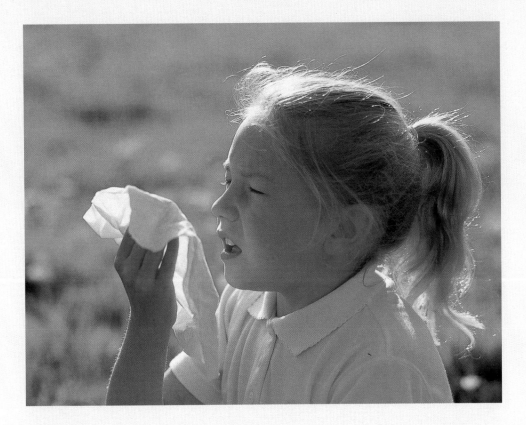

any further assumptions about you. And that just goes to emphasise the point that so little is actually known about why some people suffer from hayfever.

HOW TO USE THIS BOOK

We may not know much about why people suffer from hayfever, but we do understand the mechanisms by which the body is affected and the range of symptoms that result. This information, which is essential to a full understanding of the condition, is given in the first section of this book, 'Hayfever and conventional medicine', along with a note about conventional medical treatments and their main advantages and disadvantages.

Hayfever usually develops in the teens, but it can also attack young children.

Next, in the core of the book, is a rundown of the various alternative and natural remedies for hayfever, from nutritional techniques to hydrotherapies – all of them can play a part in relieving the symptoms of an attack, making it less likely that one will develop.

The final section of the book, 'Avoidance and prevention', shows you the common-sense steps that you can take to avoid the problem in the first place – without having to spend the spring and summer in a state of complete hibernation.

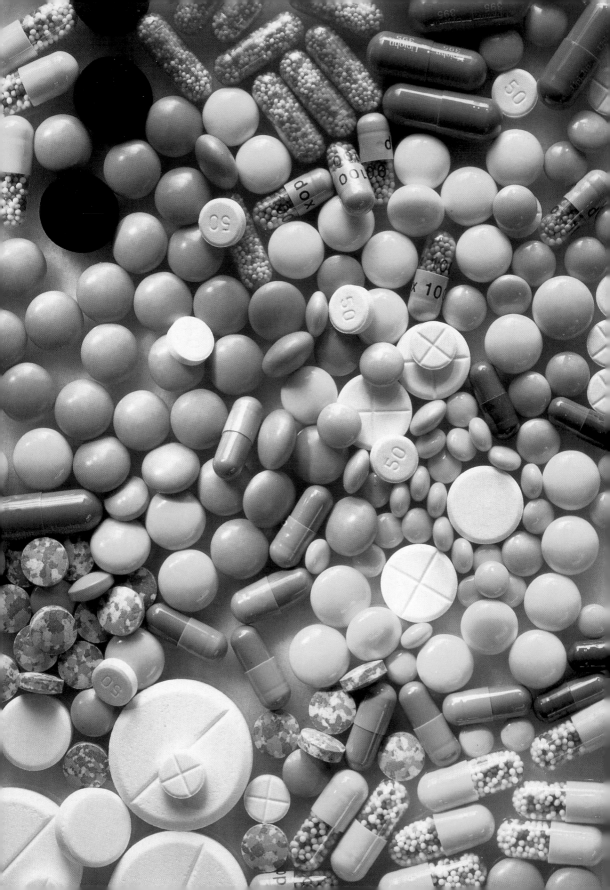

CHAPTER 1

Hayfever &
Conventional Medicine

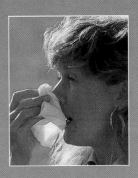

'**K**now your enemy' is a fairly sound principle in most areas of life, and it certainly holds true when it comes to dealing with hayfever. For hayfever is caused by an allergy to pollen, and an understanding of how the allergic response works and the nature of pollen is vital to an understanding of the condition itself.

Doctors often refer to hayfever as 'allergic rhinitis', because pollen is just one cause of allergic rhinitis and there are other substances to which sufferers have the same allergic response, such as hairs and skin particles from dogs and cats and droppings from mites and other insects.

In this section of the book you will find out about how pollen causes the release of special chemicals inside the body's tissues, the effects that they have on body systems and how conventional medicine tries both to prevent their release and neutralise them.

> **WHAT IS HAYFEVER? • TYPES OF POLLEN**
> **HOW POLLEN ATTACKS HUMANS • CROSS-REACTIONS**
> **OTHER ALLERGENS • OTHER FACTORS**
> **THE SYMPTOMS • GENETIC FACTORS**
> **PSYCHOLOGICAL FACTORS**
> **CONVENTIONAL MEDICAL TREATMENTS**

What is hayfever?

The simple words 'hayfever is an allergic reaction to pollen' are true enough, but they conceal an extremely complex sequence of reactions. And in order to understand how the sequence unravels, you have to understand something of the workings of the immune system: the body's natural defence mechanism against foreign invaders.

It is a bit confusing to think of the immune system as something as defined as a 'system', because in fact it is a response that takes place throughout the body. A clear fluid, known as lymph, seeps out of the blood into a network of vessels that form the lymphatic system, carrying with it millions of immune cells, to bathe all the cells in the body.

Among these immune cells are chemicals called antibodies. The body creates vast numbers of antibodies soon after birth, with each one having the capability of recognising a specific type of chemical – each type is known as an antigen. When an antibody recognises an antigen it sticks to it and acts as a marker, so that other defensive cells can find it and destroy it; at the same time, the body starts to mass-produce further quantities of the same antibody (this is the principle of vaccination, or immunisation).

Antibodies mark antigens in different ways: some markers attract immune cells that work gently over a long period of time, without any specific symptoms; but others attract special immune cells, called mast cells and basophils, that work very rapidly and viciously by releasing potent chemicals – one of which is histamine, which is also found in stinging nettles – in order to destroy the offending antigens quickly and completely. These markers are chemicals known as imunoglobulin E, or IgE.

These chemicals have a number of effects. The most obvious effect is inflammation: this causes the small blood vessels, the capillaries, to dilate; and more fluid seeps from them into the surrounding tissues, so that there is an increase in the amount of lymph fluid in the area. But these chemicals also act as a signal for more mast cells to join in the fight and release further chemicals, and more and more antibodies that are specific to the antigen are produced – so the exercise is self-perpetuating, until the invading antigens have been destroyed and the body is safe.

So far, so good. But the problem comes when the body becomes confused between what is potentially harmful, and thus an antigen, and

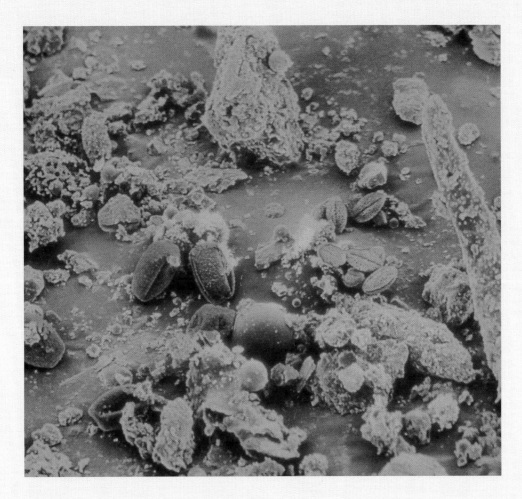

what is harmless. In cases of allergies, antibodies in those affected react as if a harmless substance is harmful – this substance is treated as an antigen, and is called an 'allergen'. In the case of hayfever, the allergen is a chemical on the surface of pollen – of course there are different chemicals on the surface of different types of pollen, which is why hayfever sufferers often react more strongly to one type of pollen than another.

As we've seen, why the body decides that a substance is an allergen is

An electron micrograph of common household allergens, including dust, pollen grains, fungal spores and mould.

something of a mystery, although a genetic factor is known to be involved (see pages 30-31). But we do know that the severity of an individual's response to the pollen allergen depends on how many IgE markers are present in that individual's body: the more there are, the more mast cells are attracted (basophils are also attracted, but it is mast cells that have the prime role in the case of hayfever). That means that more chemicals are released, which causes more inflammation and makes the symptoms of hayfever considerably worse.

PRIMING AND LATE-PHASE REACTIONS

Hayfever differs from many other allergies, in that its symptoms often become worse, day by day. There are two reasons for this. The first is a problem known as 'priming', and depends on the fact that hayfever sufferers are exposed to the pollen to which they are allergic for days at a time. If the pollen allergen was destroyed on its first appearance and there was no repeat of any exposure to it, the symptoms of hayfever might well only be a minor irritation.

By the time a second exposure of the pollen allergen occurs, millions more antibodies have been manufactured and are available to mark the allergens. This means that more mast cells arrive and more histamine is released making the hayfever symptoms more extreme. And the process is repeated the next day, with the numbers of antibodies available, and so mast cells, increasing every time there is any exposure.

To make matters worse, the nose itself becomes more sensitive to histamine (and other irritants such as cigarette smoke) during a hayfever attack. It therefore reacts with increasing violence as the attack progresses.

The second reason for the increasing severity of symptoms is something called a 'late-phase reaction'. Some of the immune cells – types called neutrophils and eosinophils – take longer to reach the site where the allergen has been detected than others. As a result, the nose of a hayfever sufferer may become inflamed once more many hours after the original symptoms have passed. The membranes of the nose become more and more sensitive as a result of the continual presence of histamine, with the result that only a small amount of the allergen is required to spark another allergic reaction.

This means that each day the scene is set for a stronger allergic reaction the next day and the amount of allergen needed to achieve that reaction goes down. So a low pollen count one day does not always mean a reduction in hayfever symptoms during that day.

The late-phase reaction also occurs in cases of asthma caused by an allergy to pollen. The bronchi are normally less sensitive and slower to respond to pollen than the nose, but once they have been affected, the late-phase reaction that follows an asthma attack leaves the bronchi inflamed and sensitive, and only a small amount of allergen is required to bring about a further attack. A continuous sequence of late-phase reactions followed by fresh attacks can leave the bronchi so highly sensitized that the asthma becomes a year-round rather than a seasonal condition.

HOW PRIMING AND LATE PHASE REACTIONS WORK

PRIMING (early reaction)

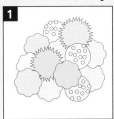
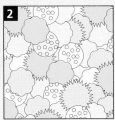
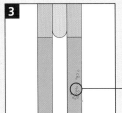
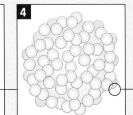

First exposure to pollen
This causes mild symptoms and creates anitbodies.

Second exposure to pollen
Antibodies are already present in abundance.

Antibodies
These bind to both pollen grains and to immune cells, mainly mast cells.

Mast cells
Thousands of antibodies cover the surface of the mast cell.

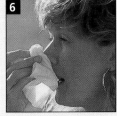
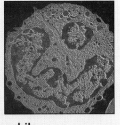

Symptoms may continue for a while and then subside. However, symptoms reappear 2-12 hours later because of a late phase reaction (see below).

Histamine
The antibodies stimulate the mast cells to release histamine.

Symptoms
Typical symptoms – itchy eyes and, runny nose – follow rapidly.

LATE PHASE (delayed reaction)

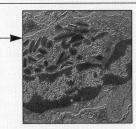
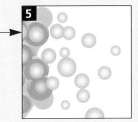
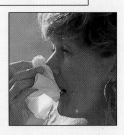

The late phase
As a result, symptoms recur a few hours after the initial attack,

Eosinophils and neutrophils
These types of immune cells arrive later at the allergen site, releasing further packets of histamine into the tissues.

sometimes combining with, and making worse, a fresh reaction to a new intake of pollen.

Types of pollen

Hayfever sufferers are often only affected by one major type of pollen, although some people react only to individual subdivisions within each type. For example, grass pollen is the main cause of hayfever in northern Europe, but a sufferer may be affected either by just one of the 12 main species of grass pollen, or by a combination of different grass pollens. Cross-reactions (see pages 20-21) are common in such people, who are hardest hit just before, during and after June, when levels of grass pollen are at their highest. In such circumstances, it is not always useful to identify the specific type of pollen that is responsible any further – just to know that grass pollen is the cause is sufficient.

A reaction to tree pollen is much the same, although the season for this differs in that it lasts from March to May. Once more, cross-reactions are common – particularly between birch and hazel trees – and a blanket identification of tree pollen as the culprit is usually all that is necessary.

The necessity to make a specific identification of the type of pollen (see pages 94-97) that is causing your

hayfever comes when an attack develops outside these months, in late summer or early autumn. In such cases, identification is much more difficult, too, because one allergy may hide another: a sensitivity to weed pollen, for example, may hide an underlying allergy to mould spores. The situation is also much less clear in America and Australia, where many pollens are present throughout the year and seasonal variations are less distinct (see pages 114-123).

FLOWER PHOBIAS
Hayfever sufferers often blame their condition on the flowers in their garden, or even those which decorate a vase in their home. It is a common misconception – usually because the pollen of a rose or a lily can be seen easily, whether on the flower itself or

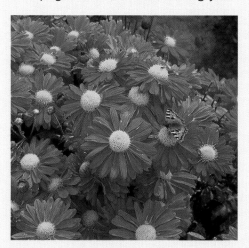

Chrysanthemums are pollinated by insects rather than wind and therefore seldom cause hayfever, except among florists.

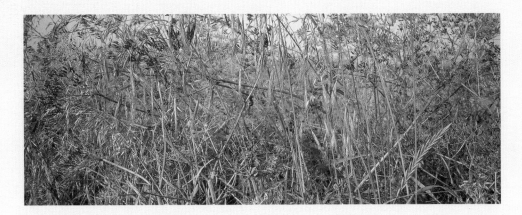

The most common cause of hayfever in early summer is wind-borne grass pollen.

on the legs of a bee – but in most cases these flowers are not actually the culprits. In fact, it is much more likely to be the pollen that cannot be seen, produced by far less showy plants, which causes a reaction.

This reaction occurs because most types of flower pollen are carried to other flowers for pollination by insects, rather than the wind. And, since such pollen forms in sticky clumps that can adhere to an insect's legs, they are generally too heavy to become airborne on their own. That is not to say that flower pollen never causes hayfever – one study has shown that around ten per cent of airborne pollen comes from insect-pollinated plants – but that it is relatively rare for it to do so.

It is far more likely that grass or tree pollen is the cause of your hayfever, since even closed buildings have been shown to contain high levels of wind-borne pollen, which the breeze has

wafted in through doors and windows from neighbouring verges, lawns and fields. Determine whether your flowers are responsible or not for your condition by making observations of whether an attack is worse when flowers are in the room or whether there is no difference.

The yellow male catkins of birch trees are laden with potentially allergenic pollen.

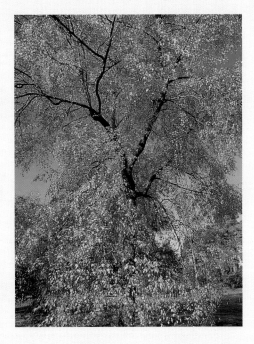

How pollen attacks humans

In order to cause an allergic reaction, pollen must enter the human tissues – nothing would happen if we just inhaled pollen and then exhaled it, or swallowed it and allowed it to pass through the digestive system.

The fact that pollen can attack human tissues – in a literal sense – depends on its prime biological function. Pollen exists to pollinate, or fertilise, other flowers. It is either carried by an insect or blown by the wind into the stigma of another flower – a stigma is a sealed entrance to a cavity deep inside the flower that contains an egg cell. Only one grain of pollen will fertilise this egg, in the same way as only one human sperm will fertilise a female egg, and it is something of a race as to which of the many pollen grains that land on a stigma will get there first.

GAUGING A PASSAGEWAY
The pollen grain is, in a sense, programmed to act aggressively to force its way through the structure of the stigma. First it releases an identifying protein – this tells the

flower on which it has landed that it is of the correct species; and it then releases protein enzymes that gauge a passageway right through the stigma. Next the pollen grain travels down this passage to meet with the egg.

The problem comes when the pollen grain is not transported to a stigma by an insect or blown to it by air currents, and instead it just rests in the air. Humans breathe in this air,

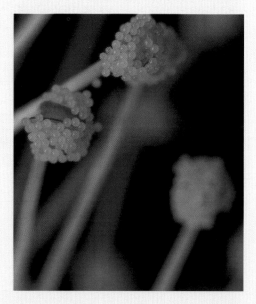

Close-up of a hibiscus flower showing the stalk like structures, known as stamens. Pollen, containing the flower's male reproductive cells is produced by the anthers at the tips of the stamens.

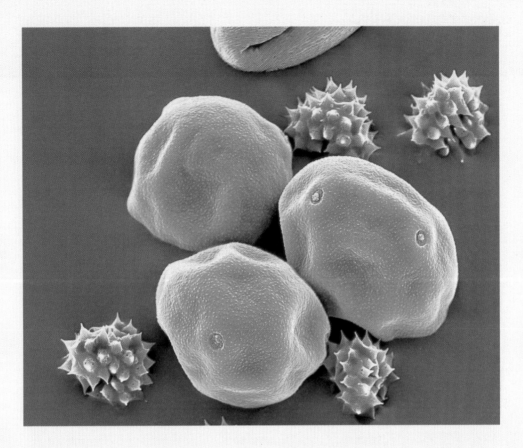

Highly magnified pollen grains of cherry (top), daisy (with spines) and hornbeam (ironwood).

and the pollen grain lodges in the membrane lining the nose. The pollen cannot distinguish the lining of the nose from the stigma of a flower, so it releases its identifying proteins, and then its enzymes. These attempt to eat their way through the nasal membrane, and infiltrate the cells of the body: the result, in those who are sensitive to these proteins and treat them as allergens, is an allergic response – hayfever. And the more grains of pollen that infiltrate the cells of the body, the more allergens there are; that means more antibodies, more mast cells, more histamine and therefore an increase in the severity of hayfever symptoms.

ACTIVE ROLE

To an extent, this response is understandable and explains why pollen is the major cause of hayfever and allergic rhinitis. For pollen is one of the few allergens which takes such an active role when it comes into contact with the tissues. In the case of dried cat saliva (see pages 22-23) and mite droppings (see pages 24-25) for example, the proteins that they contain can be treated as allergens, but they do not release chemicals that try to infiltrate cells.

Cross-reactions

We've looked at how antibodies recognise allergens (see pages 12-15), such as pollen, but it would be a mistake to think that they can identify an individual allergen with complete precision. In fact, recognition is based on fairly broad characteristics – which is just as well, because it means that the body can identify antigens (see pages 12-15) even if they mutate into a slightly different form, as bacteria, for example, often do. The trouble is that this ability means that when large amounts of antibodies are produced to combat one substance, they may start to recognise another substance as an allergen, too. This second reaction is known as a 'cross-reaction'.

Cross-reactions are most likely to occur between pollens from plants of the same botanical family, but they are not inevitable. If you are allergic to willow pollen, for example, you may develop a sensitivity to pollen from poplars because they are both from the *Salicaceae* family – but this is not always the case. (If you do, however, it's well worth looking at a botany book to see which other plants are in the same family, so that you can take steps to avoid them.) And sometimes, though much more rarely, you may have a cross-reaction to certain foods, or to chemicals in shampoos, for example, or cosmetics.

SYMPTOMS

Generally, cross-reactions have no effect other than to make a hayfever sufferer's life more miserable by prolonging an attack and making attacks more frequent during the season for the relevant pollen. Sometimes, though, they can cause serious swelling of the lips, tongue and throat or trigger an attack of asthma or hives. And, very rarely, they lead to an extremely serious condition called anaphylactic shock (see pages 28-29), which demands immediate medical intervention.

However, serious cross-reactions only develop very occasionally, but it is worthwhile being conscious of the possibility that they may occur if you suffer from hayfever, and especially so if you also have asthma attacks, since asthmatics are more at risk. The warning signs are tingling in the mouth and lips after having eaten or drunk something, and your response should be to make sure that you are in a position to call for help if your condition doesn't improve – as it almost certainly will.

Dandelions belong to the same family as ragweed, a common cause of hayfever in North America, and may themselves cause attacks in ragweed-sensitive people because of cross-reactions.

MEDICAL WATCHPOINT

Sensitivity to ragweed pollen is a common cause of hayfever, and cross-reactions to the pollen of other members of the daisy family (Compositae) to which it belongs are not uncommon. Unfortunately, both feverfew and chamomile, both of which are used in herbal medicines (see pages 50-55), are members of the daisy family, so you should avoid any preparations containing them if your hayfever is caused by ragweed.

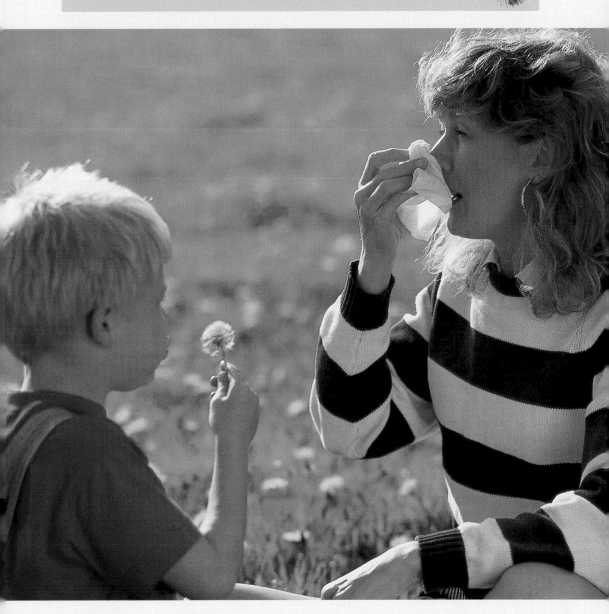

Other allergens

Although pollen is the most common cause of allergic rhinitis, which is why the condition is known as hayfever, many other allergens can be responsible for its symptoms. In fact, anything that carries protein and can be inhaled can be an allergen, and the list is long and varied. And as many of these allergens are present in the air all the year round, they can be a source of never-ending misery for those affected.

MOULD SPORES

There are far more mould spores in the air than pollen grains at any given time, but fortunately they do not give rise to strong allergic reactions in many people. Mould is a type of fungus that thrives in damp, humid conditions and, depending on the precise type of a mould its tiny spores – or seeds – may either be present in the air all year round, or be confined to a particular season. The only way to avoid them is to keep your house dry and well-aired (see pages 104-109).

CATS

It may be surprising that cats have been singled out, especially as most people think of cats as clean, fastidious animals. Indeed they are, but it is their very cleanliness that causes the problems and allergies to cats are extremely common. When a cat licks itself, tiny particles of saliva with allergenic properties dry and become airborne, eventually settling to form an invisible dust over walls, carpets, chair and curtains – this lasts for years, and can be extremely

difficult to remove. If you suffer from a cat allergy, the only real solution is to avoid them and avoid any homes in which they live, too. And although cat hairs do not carry the saliva, it will not make any difference if you replace a long-haired cat with a short-haired cat.

DOGS, HORSES AND OTHER ANIMALS

Unfortunately, people who have a tendency to allergies but live or work with animals run a fairly high risk of becoming allergic to them – whether the animal is a dog, a horse, a hamster or a guinea pig. The possibility that smaller household pets, including buderigars and canaries, might be the cause of hayfever is often overlooked, as is the allergenic potential of more unwelcome visitors such as rats and mice. Prolonged contact is not necessary for an allergy to develop. In some cases, people can be sensitised to an animal protein merely by touching someone else's clothes. Again, saliva and skin particles are the culprits, with particles of droppings also contributing to the problem.

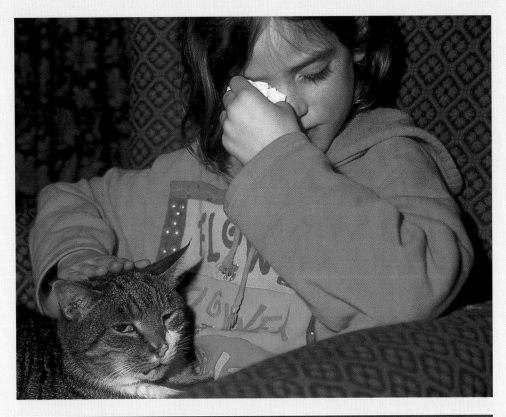

AIRBORNE PARTICLES WHICH MAY CAUSE HAYFEVER

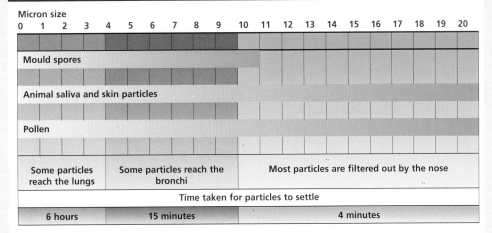

Micron size

0 1 2 3 4 5 6 7 8 9 10 11 12 13 14 15 16 17 18 19 20

Mould spores

Animal saliva and skin particles

Pollen

Some particles reach the lungs	Some particles reach the bronchi	Most particles are filtered out by the nose
Time taken for particles to settle		
6 hours	15 minutes	4 minutes

The size of a particle is a major factor in its ability to cause allergic reactions. Larger particles – 20 microns (20 thousandths of a millimetre) or more – settle rapidly in still air. Outside, however, warm air currents and winds can keep such particles as grass pollen (30 microns) aloft for considerable periods.

Other factors

You may think that your house is clean and tidy, but the unfortunate truth is that your house is almost certainly a zoo, home to millions upon millions of microscopically small creatures. All of these creatures leave minute traces, in the form of droppings or broken or dead parts of their bodies, and many of them can cause allergic rhinitis, or even asthma.

HOUSE-DUST MITES

Invisible to the naked eye, house-dust mites thrive in the warm, humid conditions of centrally heated houses. It's not a pleasant thought, but a mattress may contain as many as two million house-dust mites – during its ten-day life-cycle, a female mite can produce between 40 and 80 eggs – while sofas, curtains, carpets and cushions also house huge numbers of them. Even if you vacuum a small area of carpet for 20 minutes, using an ordinary vacuum cleaner, you will only reduce the house-dust mite population by around two per cent.

House-dust mites are scavengers, and they live on the tiny particles of dead human skin that we shed constantly. Horrible as they may sound, though, they do not cause any harm in themselves. It is their droppings that lead to the problem, because we inhale them in normal household dust, which can stay airborne for quite some time. The droppings contain a protein that is one of the house-dust mite's digestive enzymes, and it is this that is treated as an allergen by the immune system of those who are particularly sensitive.

COCKROACHES AND OTHER INSECTS

There is a tendency to think of cockroaches as an American problem. In fact, however, a recent survey in Britain found infestations of cockroaches in every part of the country. And cockroaches can give rise to allergic rhinitis in two different ways: first, allergens are found on their droppings, which are inhaled in the same way as those of house-dust mites; second, their hair, skin and wings disintegrate into minute particles, which are then inhaled. The number of cockroaches decreases in winter, so if you suffer from hayfever symptoms when you are indoors but only during the summer, it may be that it is cockroaches that are responsible for the problem.

Outdoor insects can also give rise to allergies, caused by particles on the insects' hairs or body fragments. It is unusual, although not rare, for people to be allergic to midges and

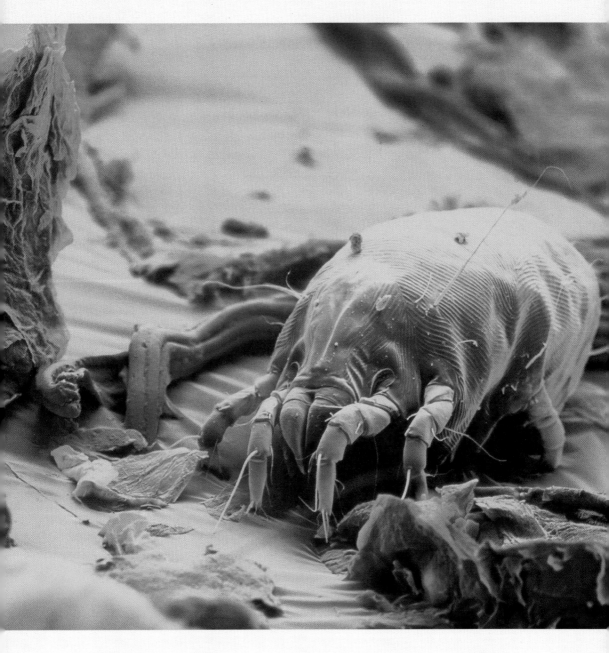

some individuals react strongly to house flies. On very rare occasions, people are allergic to bees, moths and butterflies. It has even been known for fishermen to become allergic to maggots they use as bait!

A house-dust mite under the electron microscope, feeding on skin particles in house dust. Dust mite droppings are a common cause of allergies because they are ubiquitous and because they are so small that they easily become airborne.

The symptoms

In some ways it's a little surprising that allergic rhinitis came to be called 'hayfever' when it is caused by pollen, because most hayfever sufferers never experience the high temperature and sweating characteristic of a fever. The majority of symptoms are confined to the eyes and nose, although they can progress to involve the mouth, throat, chest, sinuses and ears.

The first sign of an attack of hayfever is a tingling, itchy feeling in the eyes, nose, mouth and throat, which indicates that the body has begun to react to the presence of an allergen. In the second stage, which follows fairly quickly, the body tries to expel these foreign particles physically: the nose and eyes start to run, to flush the particles out; and then a succession of sneezes attempt to remove them more forcibly. This is something of a lost cause, however, because more particles are taken in with every breath.

While this first line of defence is being activated, antibodies are latching on to the allergens and marking them for the attention of the mast cells (see pages 12-15). These flock to the site, releasing histamine to destroy the invaders. The histamine, in turn, irritates and inflames the membranes, making them swell up. This blocks the passageways in the nose, which are already having to cope with the copious quantities of mucus that are being produced; in the case of the eyes, this inflammation may involve the membrane covering the front of the eyeball, causing conjunctivitis and leading to red, watering and very itchy eyes.

The third stage of an attack of hayfever – or of any type of allergic rhinitis – involves the spread of inflammation to other areas. The bones of the face and skull are not solid, but contain a honeycomb of cavities, called the sinuses, and mucus and, sometimes, foreign particles, can travel into the sinuses from the nose and mouth, especially when it is being produced in such cavities. This mucus may then become infected, causing further inflammation, and this increase in pressure often causes severe headaches in the forehead and aches and pains in the cheeks.

The ear often becomes involved in an attack of hayfever, too, because it is linked to the nose by means of the audito-meatory (eustachian) tube. Mucus can overflow into this tube, blocking it and giving an unpleasant sensation of tightness, because in normal circumstances this tube serves to equalise the pressure of the air inside the ear with that outside it.

And there is also a risk, especially in the case of children, that the mucus will become infected, leading to a painful condition called glue ear.

The severity of all these symptoms depends on a variety of factors: how much of the allergen you are exposed to and for how long; how frequently exposure recurs; how quickly and effectively symptoms are treated; and the nature of your individual reaction, both in physiological and emotional terms.

A nurse administers a bronchodilator drug to an infant with severe asthma.

HAYFEVER AND ASTHMA

A minority of hayfever sufferers also suffer from 'pollen asthma', a form of asthma mainly triggered by pollen, although other allergens that cause allergic rhinitis can also be responsible. The mechanism that causes the problem is not entirely clear: it may be that tiny fragments of the allergens reach the lungs by being inhaled; or, some scientists believe that an attack of hayfever makes the bronchi (the tubes that carry air to the base of the lungs) hypersensitive to other asthma triggers, such as cold air, or diesel fumes, and causes 'pollen asthma'.

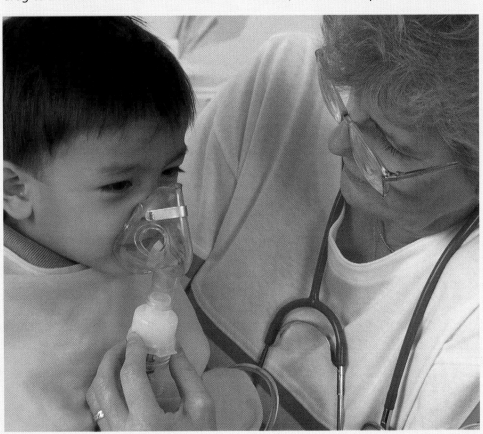

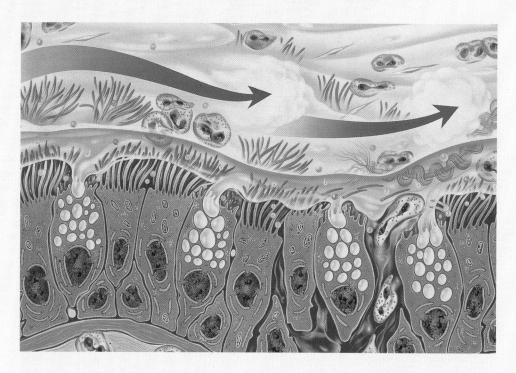

In an asthma attack, the bronchial tubes are inflamed, constricted, and covered in mucus. Drugs are inhaled to provide relief.

Whichever the case, an asthma attack is potentially a very serious event. What happens is that the muscles lining the bronchi go into spasm, making breathing wheezy and difficult in a minor attack, or almost impossible in a very serious attack. Generally, the asthmatic attacks associated with pollen asthma are not particularly significant, and the symptoms pass quickly – they can be overcome, too, by the use of breathing techniques (see pages 78-79). However, if you suffer from wheeziness, a tight chest and a dry cough from time to time you should consult your doctor, because such attacks can on occasions become considerably worse and it may be wise to have medication on hand in such cases. Many of the remedies and techniques in chapter two of this book will also make it less likely that your asthma will worsen.

ANAPHYLACTIC SHOCK
On rare occasions, sometimes as a result of a cross-reaction (see pages 20-21), an allergic reaction occurs

MEDICAL ALERT

If you have an asthma attack it is vital to stay calm and try to control your breathing using the techniques that you have practised (see pages 78-79). Sit upright, supporting your arms so that your ribs can move easily, and call for medical assistance if you are in doubt about your condition.

that is so extreme that it affects the whole body. Mast cells release all of their histamine, which dilates blood vessels to such an extent that the pressure of blood in the system falls to the point at which life can no longer be sustained. And this reaction can happen extremely quickly.

The first signs are the tingling itchiness of the nose, eyes and mouth that mark the start of the majority of allergic reactions. However, in this case, the lips and tongue are likely to swell up quickly, obstructing breathing, and the pulse will start to drop. If you think that this may be happening to you, call for an ambulance immediately. If you know that you are at risk – as many of those with serious food allergies or an allergy to wasp or insect stings are – you may well have been given a syringe of adrenaline to use in such circumstances. If so, inject it without any delay.

THE RECOVERY POSITION

The recovery position is used to avoid the dangers that can occur during unconsciousness, and ensures that the airway is open and clear.

Kneeling to one side of the victim, turn his/her head towards you and tuck the arm nearest to you under the victim's body. Lay the other arm across the victim's chest and place the ankle farthest from you over the other ankle.

Grasping the clothing over the hip farthest from you, pull the victim on to his/her front, using your knees to support the body and your hand to protect the head as you do so. Push the victim's head back to ensure a clear airway and check his/her breathing.

On the side to which the victim's face is turned, bend the arm and leg into right angles (see below). Check the position is stable and and ensure the airway is clear. Do not leave the victim unattended and wait for professional help.

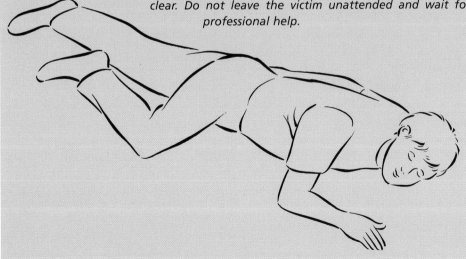

Genetic factors

Many doctors believe that the study of genetics and the manipulation of genes in genetic medicine represents the way forward for conventional medicine. This may well be the case, but at the moment the role that inherited genes plays in hayfever is far from being fully understood.

There are certain facts that are known about inherited genes. First is that it is not so much hayfever that is inherited but a tendency to allergies as a whole. The key is in the levels of immunoglobulin E (IgE) in the blood – these are the markers released by antibodies when they encounter an allergen (see pages 12-15) to attract the histamine-producing mast cells.

About a third of people have IgE levels that are sufficiently high enough to cause allergies. They are said to be 'atopic'. However, not all atopic people develop allergies – as few as one in three actually do so – and it is common for several members of a family to be atopic but with only one or two of them displaying allergic symptoms. It is probable that there are genes that decrease susceptibility to allergens as well as genes that increase it. Even in the case of identical twins, with exactly the same genetic make-up and the same environmental influences in childhood, it can happen that one twin becomes allergic while the other does not. Clearly, the development of an allergy is not a matter of simple genetic inheritance, and must involve a malfunction in several aspects of the immune system.

Taking this fact into account, there is still a 30 to 35 per cent chance that a child will develop an allergy if one parent has an allergy – whatever it may be – and a 50 to 60 per cent chance if both parents have allergies. And as one child in six develops an allergy even when there is no family history of allergies or hayfever, this means that the chances of developing an allergy are doubled in the first case and quadrupled in the latter.

The question is: 'Which allergy will it be?' There is only a very slightly higher chance that the allergy will cause hayfever: it could be to peanuts, for example, or to cow's milk. And even then, allergies can change – it is not uncommon for children to lose an allergy as they grow up, only to become allergic to something else. (One factor that is thought to have some effect here is the antigens to which the child is exposed, and becomes sensitised to, in early life.)

GENETIC FACTORS – YOUR SUSCEPTIBILITY TO HAYFEVER

PARENTS	PARENTS	PARENTS
both with an allergy	One with an allergy	with no allergy

CHILD	CHILD	CHILD
has a 50-60% chance of developing an allergy	has a 30-35% chance of developing an allergy	has a 15% chance of developing an allergy

The likelihood that you will develop hayfever – or another allergy – is considerably increased if there is a family history of the condition. However, a child's environment in the first few months of life is also thought to be important and protection for a susceptible newborn infant from, for example, grass pollen, may well be important.

This information leads us to one of the theories about why the incidence of allergies, including hayfever, is rising so fast in the West whereas allergies are rare in the Third World. The explanation, some people believe, is quite simply that the hygiene, sterility and vaccinations that are part of modern life in developed countries leave the immune system with little to do. As a result, it over-reacts, turning the aggressive mast cells and basophils (see pages 12-15) on to minor irritants, rather than the serious infections they were designed to combat.

WORKING OUT YOUR HISTORY

It's well worth recording any family history of allergies – not just to hayfever, but to anything, and not forgetting the extended family as well as your mother and father.

Note down, too, whether you had any childhood allergies – again, record any allergies, not just those that may have caused allergic rhinitis – or eczema.

Next, write down what you can remember of your past attacks of hayfever: how old were you when you first had one?; do you have attacks at at particular times of the year?; do you have attacks throughout the year?; does an attack correlate with any particular circumstance?

All of this information will not only help you to establish the beginnings of a pattern to your attacks, but it will be invaluable to any doctor who tries to identify the substance to which you are allergic, or confirm your identification of it.

Psychological factors

People tend to object when you say that psychological factors are involved in the majority of medical conditions – they think that you're saying: 'It's all in the mind.' And it isn't, of course. Nevertheless, it is a fact that stress – worry, mental and emotional pressure – plays an important part in both the cause of and the response to numerous medical problems, and hayfever is among them.

One study showed that children whose parents are aggressive and quick-tempered, and emotionally closed and over-protective, suffer more attacks of hayfever, with worse symptoms, than children who live in a calm, peaceful home environment. To appreciate why this should be so, it's important to understand how the stress reaction works.

THE EFFECTS OF STRESS

It is only in recent times, in terms of our evolutionary history, that human beings have not had to live their daily lives under the threat of extreme physical danger. As a result, we retain the primitive systems that enabled primitive humans to survive, and these can be summed up in the 'fight or flight' reaction. Essentially, this means that danger – the approach of a sabre-toothed tiger, for example – would trigger an immediate response by the involuntary, or autonomic nervous system, without any conscious thought. Stress hormones – adrenaline being one of the most important – flood the body, raising the heartbeat, increasing the rate of breathing, in order to increase oxygen levels, raising blood pressure, and diverting blood and the nutrients it carries away from inessential systems such as the digestion and into the muscles. In short, the body is prepared for decisive action.

Our primitive human then has a choice: he or she can either fight, or run away. In either case the situation is resolved quickly, and the body can return to normal. Unfortunately this 'fight or flight' response is also triggered, though at a lower level, by emotional stress, and there is no swift resolution to the problem. This means that stress hormones are ever-present in the body, raising blood pressure, increasing muscular tension and maintaining high levels of blood sugar.

STRESS AND HAYFEVER

As far as hayfever is concerned, this reaction has two effects. The first is that the adrenal glands, which produce adrenaline, are working full-time and are unable to produce sufficient extra adrenaline to fight the histamine that is released by mast

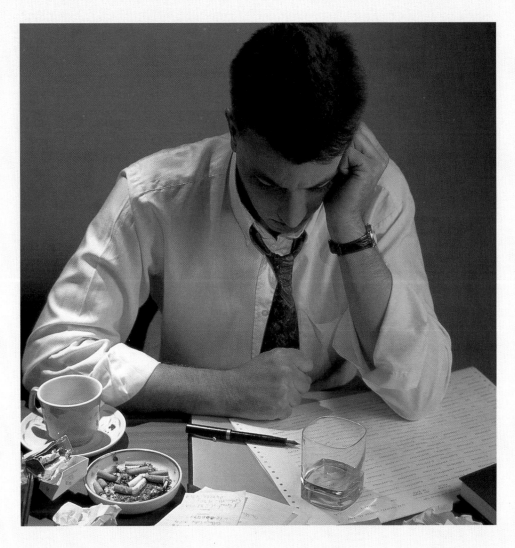

cells (see pages 12-15). The second relies on the fact there are two parts to the autonomic nervous system: the sympathetic system, which primarily controls the stress response; and the parasympathetic system – it is this that deals with the immune response and the fight against infection and foreign bodies. And if the autonomic system as a whole is constantly active, monitoring the stress response, the immune response is likely to suffer.

Stress, depression, anxiety – all can play a part in triggering an allergy. Hayfever is less affected by psychological factors than asthma, but it is still important to retain a positive attitude towards the condition.

It is for this reason that some of the remedies discussed in the next section of this book are concerned with reducing stress and emphasising a positive approach to dealing with the symptoms of hayfever.

Conventional medical treatments

Since the detailed mechanism of how an allergic reaction works is still uncertain, conventional medical treatments generally aim to relieve symptoms by the use of drugs rather than effect a lasting cure. Here we describe how these drugs work and what their side-effects can, on occasions, be. However the intention here is not to dissuade you from taking any such drugs – and you should certainly take them if they have been prescribed by your doctor.

The only medical alternative to drugs is desensitisation treatment (see pages 36-37), which is time-consuming and not without dangers – it can occasionally, for example, trigger off the allergic reaction it is intended to prevent. Conventional treatments are more successful in treating the symptoms of hayfever than in dealing with the underlying cause.

As far as short-term remedies are concerned, the drugs used fall into four categories, which are used singly or in combination: antihistamines; sympathomimetics; corticosteroids; and mast cell stabilisers.

ANTIHISTAMINES AND SYMPATHOMIMETICS

Since it is histamine, released by the mast cells (see pages 12-15), that causes most of the symptoms in hayfever, it would seem to make sense to counter the effects of histamine with a drug specifically designed for that purpose. And antihistamines, which work by moving histamine molecules away from receptors to which they would otherwise bind, certainly do the job effectively – although they have no impact on a blocked nose. You can buy them over the counter at most pharmacy stores, and it is often helpful if you take a course of them just before the hayfever season starts.

The trouble is that antihistamines have their downside, too. Some of the older types of histamine can make you feel drowsy, but, variously, there is also the possibility of dizziness, tremors and blurred vision – for this reason, you should never drive while taking antihistamines. This is less of a problem with the most recent generation of antihistamines but the problem still exists. In addition, antihistamines should

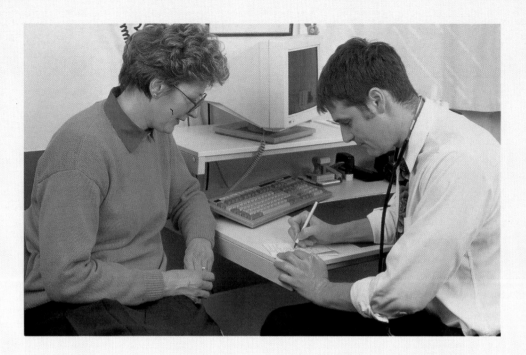

A doctor can often help to identify the cause of an allergy, as well as prescribing drugs to alleviate the symptoms.

not be taken in a number of other circumstances (see Medical Watchpoint, page 37).

Sympathomimetics mock the action of adrenaline, which counteracts histamine naturally inside the body. These drugs, many of which can be bought over the counter are normally take in the form of nose or eye drops, and are effective at unblocking the nose – acting like adrenaline, they force the blood vessels in the nose to contract, so reducing the swelling, and have a similar effect when used on red eyes. Again, unfortunately, there are a few disadvantages: first, adrenaline is one of the stress hormones, so sympathomimetics can induce the 'flight or flight' reaction (see pages 32-33) to a degree, with all this entails; second, if they are taken for longer than a few weeks the nose will come accustomed to them and large doses will be necessary, which in turn will increase the side-effects.

To give the benefits of both types of drugs – but the problems and side-effects, too – antihistamines and sympathomimetics are sometimes both included in some preparations. These can be bought over the counter, and come in the form of either liquid or tablets.

CORTICOSTEROIDS
One of the main problems caused by allergic rhinitis is inflammation, and corticosteroids are anti-inflammatory drugs that mimic the effect of cortisol, a hormone produced naturally by the

body. They are powerful drugs, and must be prescribed by a doctor, but they work effectively, and can be given in a variety of ways. The most common of these is in the form of nose drops, though corticosteroid eye drops can also alleviate conjunctivitis; they can also be given in the form of tablets or in a single, slow-release injection that lasts for the whole hayfever season.

This time the disadvantage is that that cortisol, which corticosteroids mimic, has a significant effect on the chemical balance of the body and corticosteroids can add to this effect, to the detriment of this chemical balance. Another possibility is that the body produces less cortisol, with equally detrimental effects, because of the presence of the artificial corticosteroids. However, corticosteroid drugs are changed synthetically to boost the anti-inflammatory effect and reduce the effect on the body's chemistry, and it is fair to say – in the case of nose and eye drops at least – that any detrimental effect is minimal. The problems are only likely to arise in the case of an extended course of tablets or a slow-release injection.

MAST CELL STABILISERS
Corticosteroids themselves have a certain amount of success when it comes to stabilising mast cells (see pages 12-15) and reducing the amount of histamine that they release. Recently, however, several drugs have been developed that have

this specific task – the best-known is *sodium cromoglycate*. These have no major side-effects, though there may be some slight irritation of the nasal membranes, and in some cases they have been known to actually trigger an attack of asthma or an allergic reaction. However, such instances are rare, and it is well worth asking your doctor if you can try mast cell stabilisers as they may work for you. They are available as eye drops or nose drops, and can be bought over the counter. It is well worth starting a course of mast cell stabilisers several weeks before the start of the pollen season.

DESENSITISATION THERAPY
There are three types of desensitisation therapy, the only treatment that attempts to cure hayfever in the long term: hypo-sensitisation, enzyme-potentiated desensitisation and neutralisation.

Hyposensitisation involves injecting a series of solutions of a given allergen beneath the skin: at first the solution is extremely dilute, but its strength is increased, week by week over a period of ten weeks or so – the idea is to allow the body to learn to tolerate the allergen. This treatment has to be repeated before each pollen season for four or five years, so it is very time-consuming, Nevertheless it is often successful. However, it is now extremely difficult to obtain this form of treatment outside of special hayfever centres, of which there are few (see pages 124-126). This is because there is a significant risk that those treated will develop anaphylactic shock (see pages 28-29). In practical terms, this form of treatment is only now available to a very few.

Enzyme-potentiated desensitisation (EPD), however, is more widely available and is successful in around 50 per cent of cases. A collection of various different pollens and allergens is mixed with a special enzyme – a chemical that can act as a catalyst to other chemical reactions – and injected beneath the skin to desensitise the body to the allergens. Treatment is given before the hayfever season starts, and may have to be repeated for as long as five years, depending on the patient.

Neutralisation therapy relies on injecting allergens beneath the skin or placing drops of a solution of allergens under the tongue: various concentrations are used, until no allergic reaction can be detected – this concentration is said to represent the patient's 'neutralising dose'. A solution of this strength is made up, and the patient is asked to take two to three drops a day at the beginning of the pollen season, reducing the dose thereafter.

MEDICAL WATCHPOINT

Do not take antihistamines if:

- *it is essential that you drive*
- *you are taking any other medication and have not asked your doctor whether it is wise to take them*
- *you have any heart or circulatory problems or high blood pressure*
- *you have any liver, kidney or urinary problems*

Do not take sympathomimetics, either on their own or in combination with antihistamines, if:

- *you have heart or circulatory problems or high blood pressure*
- *you are pregnant, trying to become pregnant or breast-feeding*
- *you have epilepsy*
- *you are taking any other medication and have not asked your doctor whether it is wise to take them*

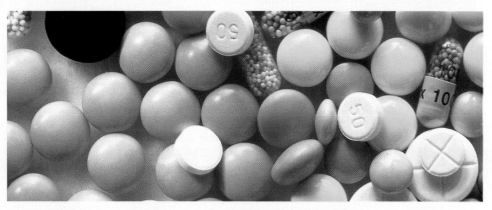

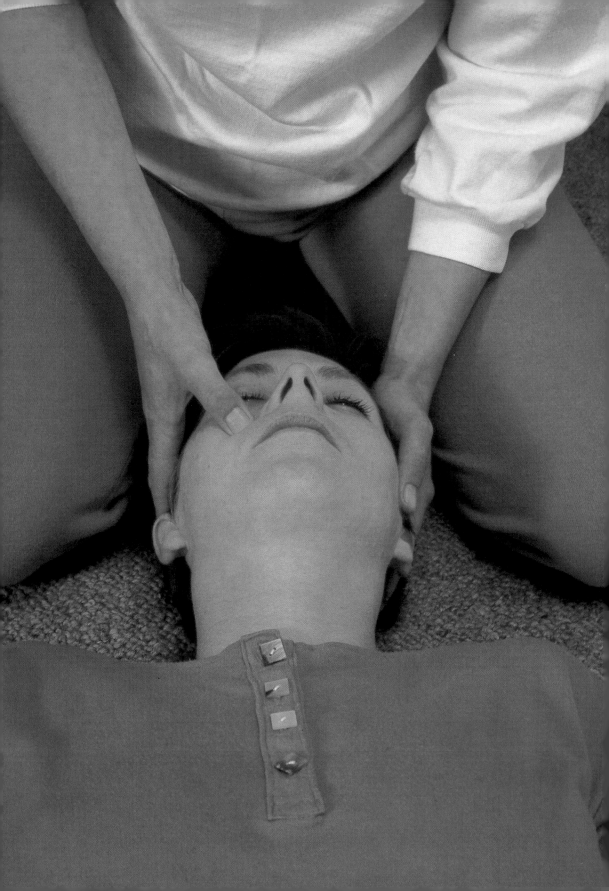

CHAPTER 2

Alternative Treatments &
Natural Remedies

Now that you know how hayfever works, it is easier to see what can be done to treat the condition, preventively and during an attack. Alternative treatments and natural remedies concentrate on boosting the body's immune system so that the allergens can be destroyed, with symptoms being kept to a minimum; counteracting the symptoms of hayfever by the use of natural antihistamines; and holistically keeping the various systems of the body in balance and stress-free. This chapter shows how the body's natural healing abilities can be harnessed to reduce the misery of hayfever.

DIET & NUTRITION • NATUROPATHY • HOMEOPATHY
HERBAL REMEDIES • BACH FLOWER REMEDIES
MASSAGE & AROMATHERAPY • ACUPUNCTURE
ACUPRESSURE • REFLEXOLOGY
RELAXATION & EXERCISE • BREATHING TECHNIQUES
POSTURE • THE ALEXANDER TECHNIQUE
VISUALISATION • SELF-HYPNOSIS & HYPNOTHERAPY
HYDROTHERAPY

Diet & nutrition

Many people believe that one reason why the number of people suffering from allergies – and from hayfever in particular – has increased is that our immune system no longer develops properly. As a result of this, the body does not possess a sufficient number of the antibodies that can attract cells that work gently, over a period (see pages 12-15), to destroy antigens, and so help is needed from the more aggressive mast cells, which cause hayfever or allergy symptoms.

One culprit for this lack of development of the immune system is thought to be vaccinations, but another is our dependence on refined foods. Therefore dietary and nutritional measures can help the immune system to develop properly and boost the level of the antibodies that help destroy allergens without giving rise to symptoms. In addition, they can also significantly help to reduce the severity of symptoms.

FOODS TO AVOID

Here is a list of foods to avoid, either because they depress the immune system, increase the chances of an attack of hayfever or make the symptoms of hayfever much worse.

Dairy products

It is advisable to reduce the amount of dairy products, such as eggs, milk, and cheese, that you consume during the spring and summer as they increase the body's ability to produce mucus and catarrh. Cow's milk, in particular, should be avoided – switch to soya milk instead.

Sugar and wheat

Grass pollens all come from the same botanical family as sugar and wheat which are a common cause of allergic reactions, so it is worthwhile cutting down on them in your daily diet.

Refined carbohydrates

Research has shown that refined carbohydrates depress the immune system within an hour of being eaten. White bread, sweets, cake, biscuits and chocolate are all refined carbohydrates and are best avoided by hayfever sufferers.

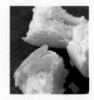

Animal fats

The effects of animal fats on the body's immune system is not completely certain, but it is thought that a diet that is high in animal fats can reduce the immune system's efficiency. Therefore it would be wise to limit the amount of animal fats in your diet.

MEDICAL WATCHPOINT

Growing children need plenty of calcium to build their bones, and women after the menopause and the elderly both require calcium to guard against osteoporosis, or brittle bones. Dairy products are one of the main sources of calcium, so if you are one of the people who are allergic to dairy produce, or it intensifies your hayfever symptoms and therefore cut down on dairy products it may be advisable to take a calcium supplement every day – please seek medical advice.

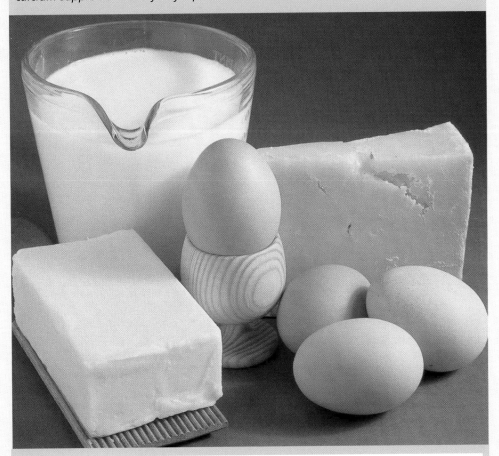

IMMUNE SYSTEM SUPPRESSORS

There are many reasons why you should not smoke and avoid alcohol, and caring for your immune system is just one of them. Alcohol and smoking both deplete the body's store of the B vitamins and zinc, both of which are vital if the immune system is to function properly. Additionally, alcohol's effect on the liver inhibits the production of a chemical that helps break down histamine, so if you drink alcohol your hayfever symptoms are likely to persist for longer.

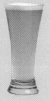

FOODS TO CHOOSE

The list that follows contains foods that are good for you and will help to boost the immune system, thus helping you to combat your hayfever symptoms. Vitamins B5 (pantothenic acid), B6 and C are all natural anti-histamines, as are magnesium and folic acid. In addition, vitamins B, C and E, taken together with an adequate supply of protein, help promote a healthy immune system. So choose a balanced diet that contains an adequate amount of all these ingredients.

Zinc

This useful mineral is essential for the proper functioning of the body's immune system. It is contained in the following foods: crabmeat, oysters, white turkey meat, baked potato skins, shellfish, pulses, cottage cheese, bran, milk and red meats.

Magnesium

A natural antihistamine, this mineral plays a vital role in many aspects of the body's chemistry, including the immune system. An increased intake of magnesium has been shown to reduce the frequency and severity of hayfever attacks. It can be found in the following foods: nuts, winkles, shrimps, soya beans and fresh, green, leafy vegetables (the darker green the better).

Vitamin B5

Also known as pantothenic acid, this vitamin is valuable in combating excess histamine. It can be found in: eggs, whole grain cereals and white meat.

Vitamin B6

This vitamin is essential in the processing of several vital chemicals required by the immune system. It is contained in the following foods: kidney beans, chicken, sunflower seeds, tuna, spinach, pulses and rice.

Vitamin B Group: Folic Acid

Another member of the vitamin B group, folic acid is essential for the functioning of the central nervous system, and is very important for health in the vulnerable years of early childhood. It can be found in the following foods: liver, kidneys, yeast, chick-peas, orange juice, soya beans, spinach, broccoli, cabbage, cauliflower, beetroot, pulses, bananas, and other fresh fruit and vegetables.

Vitamin C

This vitamin is involved in many chemical processes in the body. It is a powerful antioxidant – a group of chemicals which boost the immune system – and helps in the production of important hormones. It is contained in the following foods: broccoli, cabbage, citrus fruits, spinach, tomatoes, bananas, carrots and all fresh fruit and vegetables.

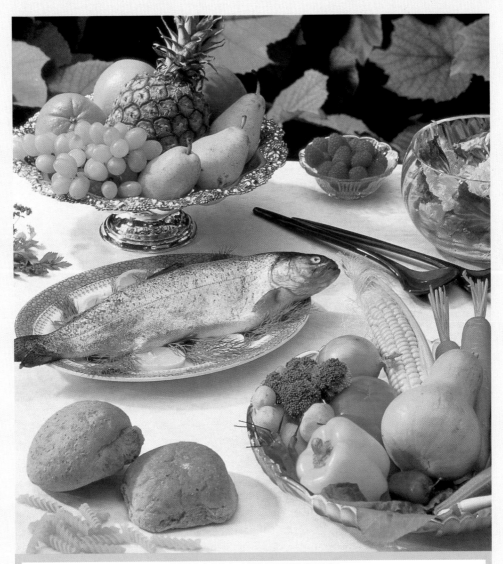

MEDICAL WATCHPOINT

Consult your doctor before making any sudden, major change in your diet, and be careful that you do not overdose on vitamin supplements – some vitamins can be harmful in excess. You should be able to acquire all of the vitamins that you need in a balanced, healthy diet, so all that you will need is a daily multi-vitamin pill.

If you are taking iron supplements – because you are pregnant, for example, or you have anaemia – you should not take zinc supplements or eat an excessive amount of foods that contain it unless asked to do so by your doctor: one affects the absorption of the other.

Naturopathy

Naturopaths believe that nature is the best healer of disease, and that symptoms are an expression of the body's fight against any imbalance within it in an attempt to recover homeostasis, or equilibrium. The imbalance that is causing the problem is the result of what naturopaths consider to be an 'unnatural' lifestyle: toxins build up in the body as a result of a bad diet, inadequate exercise and stress.

Naturopathy is an ancient therapy – it goes back at least as far as the days of Hippocrates, the physician of Ancient Greece – and the homeostasis that it stresses is a similar concept to that of the *prana* of Ayurvedic medicine and the *chi* (life energy), or yin and yang, of Chinese medicine.

You can put the basic principles of preventive naturopathy into practice at home – the rules are commonsense. To counter a build-up of toxins, remain healthy and prevent an attack of hayfever you should make sure that you breathe fresh air, drink clean water, eat wholesome food, and take adequate exercise and rest.

TAKING ACTION

However, naturopaths believe that once a condition has developed more active measures are needed. These are aimed not at relieving symptoms – which, after all, are only the body's outward signs of an attempt to rid itself of toxins – but at encouraging the body's own healing systems to flush the toxins out. In fact, the symptoms are considered a healthy sign, because they show that the body is fighting the toxins and should be encouraged to do so – in much the same way that getting up a sweat helps to cure a fever. Any aggressive treatment would put the body under more stress, and make things worse, naturopaths believe, so they stress that the treatment should be gentle, and take into account the whole person, considering his or her mental state and environment.

Naturopaths often advocate short fasts of two to three days, during which only vegetable and fruit juices are consumed, to allow the body time to rest, in a physiological sense, and to boost the immune system in order to fight any toxins. They believe, too,

MEDICAL WATCHPOINT

Do not attempt to fast for longer than two days unless you have consulted your doctor beforehand. Do not stop taking any medically prescribed drugs without consultation, this is especially important if you have any pre-existing medical condition.

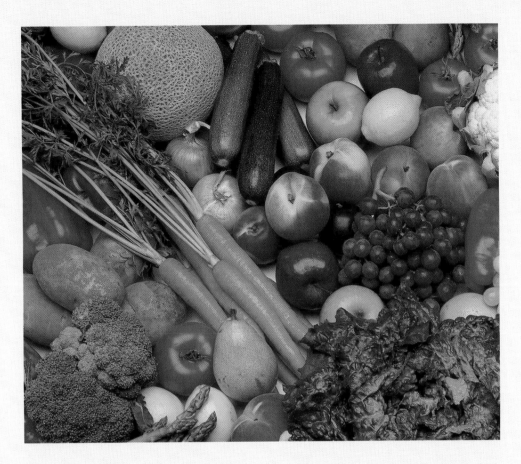

that many modern ailments are the result of poor function of the bowels, and some naturopaths advocate the use of colonic irrigation. This practice can be dangerous, however, and the majority of naturopaths suggest colonic cleansing instead: the use of a high-fibre dietary supplement that has a similar result and is safer and cheaper. After treatment, they stress the importance of a diet that is rich in unrefined foods and fibre.

CONSULTING A NATUROPATH

In some countries, such as Germany, naturopaths have a similar standing to doctors and recommend that a

Naturopathy stresses the importance of a natural, organic, chemical-free diet, with a high fibre content.

number of treatments are tried alongside their own, such as hydrotherapy, herbalism, acupuncture, massage, chiropractice and homeopathy. Recognition for naturopathy lags behind in some other western countries, but most now have recognised three- to four-year courses of study in the subject, which lead to a diploma or a degree. Contact the appropriate national organisation to find the name of a qualified naturopath in your area (see pages 124-126).

Homeopathy

Some 200 years ago, Samuel Hahnemann, a German physician and chemist, analysed the results of his observations and of experiments on himself and came up with 'The Law of Similars'. This states that a remedy can cure a disease if it produces symptoms similar to those of the disease in a healthy person. This theory became the groundstone of what was to be homeopathy.

The trouble with 'The Law of Similars' theory was that the use of such remedies caused inevitable side-effects, since they triggered symptoms. However, after further experiment, Hahnemann found that a considerable dilution of the remedy not only eliminated side-effects, but made the remedy more effective: he had discovered the principle of the 'Minimum Dose', and called the way in which it worked 'potentisation'.

Today, homeopathic medicine is well-established world-wide, and its efficacy is accepted by many practitioners of conventional medicine. It is not just used as a treatment for specific conditions, but as a general strengthening agent for the immune system, so homeopathic treatments can be used as an effective preventive measure against hayfever. However, choosing the correct treatment for hayfever involves a number of factors, and is best undertaken on a long-term basis by a qualified homeopath.

HOMEOPATHY FOR HAYFEVER

There are two specific homeopathic treatments for hayfever: *Euphrasia* (eyebright) and *Allium cepa* (red onion) – the use of onion as a homeopathic remedy is understandable when you consider what happens when you cut an onion: your eyes start to stream, just as in hayfever. Both can be bought at health stores, although you will also need to buy a few bottles of lactose (milk sugar) carrier pills, some pure alcohol, a test-tube stand and test-tubes and a pipette. The next step is to make up the remedies, by dilution and re-dilution (see opposite page), which as well as increasing their effect, ensures that they can be given to anyone, of any age, without danger.

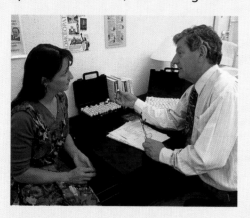

Consulting a homeopathic practitioner.

MAKING A HOMEOPATHIC REMEDY

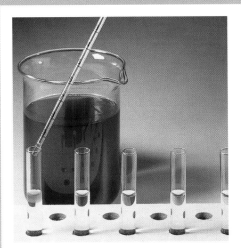

The first step is to produce a 'tincture', by soaking the plant material (either *Euphrasia* or *Allium cepa*) in pure alcohol for a few weeks. Once this 'mother tincture' is ready, it is time to start diluting the tincture to the correct potency.

For hayfever remedies, it should be '6x' – meaning that it has been diluted six times, each dilution being in a ratio of one drop of the previous liquid to nine drops of pure alcohol. After each dilution, the mixture is shaken vigorously by knocking it against the palm of the hand – 'succussation'.

MAKING A 6X POTENCY

1 Making sure that the remedy is of the correct potency is not a difficult procedure, but accuracy is required. First of all, set six test tubes up in a rack, and fill each of them with nine drops of pure alcohol. Have your pipette ready and a bottle of lactose (milk sugar) carrier pills at hand.

2 Measure one drop – of the same size used for the drops of alcohol – of the mother tincture and place it in the first test-tube: you now have a 1x potency remedy.

3 Succuss the liquid to mix it thoroughly by knocking the test-tube against the palm of your hand.

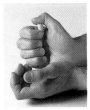

4 Place one drop of the 1x mixture from the first tube into the second tube, and succuss again. Repeat the process with the next four tubes.

5 Now at 6x potency, the mixture can be added to the bottle of lactose carrier pills, and the homeopathic remedy is complete.

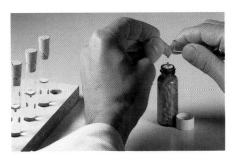

Taking the remedies

Homeopathy practice stresses that only one remedy should be taken at a time, so choose whether *Allium cepa* (red onion) or *Euphrasia* (eyebright) is the most appropriate for the symptoms that are predominant in you and try that first.

Allium cepa (red onion)

Try this remedy, at 6x potency, when:

- you sneeze frequently

- you have a heavy, burning discharge from the nose

- your eyes secrete a bland, watery fluid

- the smell of flowers aggravates the symptoms

Dosage: one dose every two to four hours for two days, then reduce the dosage to three times daily for a further three to five days.

Euphrasia (eyebright)

Try this remedy, at 6x potency, when:

- your eyes are red, burning, watery and itchy; any nasal discharge is bland

- your symptoms become worse in sunlight and the warmth, and worse in open air

Dosage: one dose every two to four hours for two days, then reduce to three times daily for a further three to five days.

Euphrasia (eyebright) can also be taken externally, in the form of eyedrops. Use drops of the mother tincture (see page 47) for this purpose.

Storing homeopathic remedies

Homeopathic remedies will keep well if you observe some basic precautions:

- they can be spoiled by heat and light, so store them in the dark, away from heat, and try to touch them as little as possible

- keep them away from any strong-smelling products, such as perfume, mothballs and massage and aromatherapy oils

- never put remedies in old containers, because traces of any original remedy will adhere to them

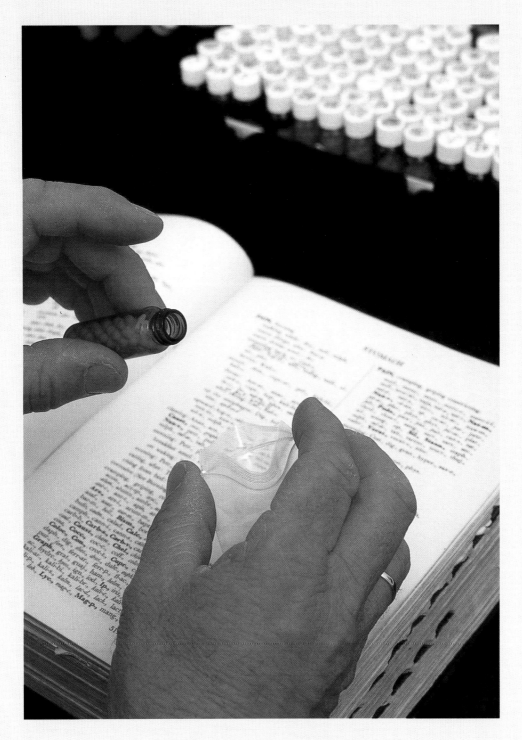

Homeopathic remedies for hayfever provide long-term prevention and short-term relief.

Herbal remedies

We know from the records that they have left behind that herbal medicine was practised by the ancient Egyptians, Romans and Greeks, but herbs were almost certainly used for healing purposes for many thousands of years before that. Today, herbal medicine is enjoying something of a revival, as people are starting to become suspicious of laboratory-produced synthetic drugs, with their risk of side-effects, and prefer the idea of using more natural substances. And, after all, the potential toxicity of herbs has been tested not in short-term laboratory tests, but over many centuries of use.

Herbal remedies certainly have a part to play in the treatment of hayfever, both in preventing and relieving the symptoms of an attack. However, preventive treatments are best prescribed by an experienced herbalist, who will draw up a picture of every aspect of your life, past and present, before deciding which preparations would be best for you.

Therefore these pages are solely concerned with the use of herbal remedies to relieve symptoms – you should consult a herbalist to obtain an appropriate course of preventive treatment.

TEAS, TINCTURES, SYRUPS AND INHALATIONS

A variety of herbs can be used to relieve the streaming eyes, runny nose, sinusitis and build-up of mucus that are characteristic of hayfever, and individual recipes for their use are given later. Some herbs act more effectively when taken in a specific way, and in the case of hayfever there are three methods of administration: in teas and tinctures; in syrups; or by inhalation.

MAKING A HERBAL TEA

Drinking tea is natural to most of us, and it's a refreshing way of taking a herbal remedy – one that makes the herb easy to assimilate and digest.

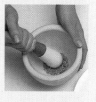

1 Chop either fresh or dried herbs finely, and blend in a pestle and mortar. Warm a teapot, and boil a kettle of water – use tap water if you have a good supply, or mineral water otherwise.

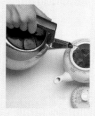

2 Add the boiling water to the teapot, cover and allow to rest for 1-3 minutes in the case of flowers, 2-4 minutes if you are using leaves and 4-10 minutes for the use of seeds, bark and hard roots.

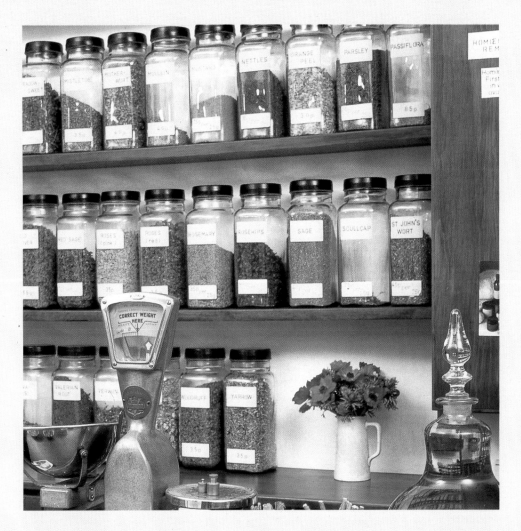

3 Strain the liquid into a cup. Do not add milk as it tends to suppress the flavour of herbal teas, but a spoonful of honey or a few drops of lemon juice can enhance the flavour.

Dosage: one cup three to six times a day, depending on the severity of symptoms. Pause to inhale the aroma before drinking, because this in itself has healing properties.

The herbalist's dispensary hasn't changed over the centuries though, today, prepared infusions and capsules are easier to find.

MEDICAL WATCHPOINT

Be alert to the possibility that some herbs may cause a cross-reaction (see pages 20-21) with certain types of pollen, especially if they come from the same group of plants. Do not use any herbs that are closely related to any plants to which you are allergic.

MAKING A TINCTURE

You may not have the time to make a herbal tea, but you can always make a herbal tincture and carry a bottle of it around with you. Traditionally, tinctures are made with alcohol, but if you do not wish to take alcohol add the dose to a quarter of a cup of water and leave it uncovered for a few hours, so the alcohol evaporates.

1 Chop or bruise the herb – to make 200-300 ml (7-10 fl oz) of tincture you will need 15 g ($\frac{1}{2}$ oz) of dried herbs, or 30 g (1 oz) of fresh herbs.

2 Put the herbs into a large jar and add a mixture of 200 ml (7 fl oz) of alcohol, such as vodka or brandy, and 85 ml (3 fl oz) of water. Seal the jar, label it and leave to stand in a cool, dark place for two weeks, turning it upside-down daily.

3 Strain the mixture through a loose-weave cotton cloth placed in a strainer, and discard the spent herbs. Then pour the strained liquid into clean, glass bottles – preferably amber ones – and label them. The tincture will keep indefinitely.

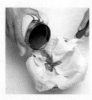

Dosage: one teaspoon three to six times a day, depending on the severity of symptoms.

MAKING A SYRUP

Syrups are the basis of many cough remedies, and generally help to thin out mucus and open up the airways.

1 Chop 40 g (1$\frac{1}{2}$ oz) of herbs and place in a pan with 900 ml (1$\frac{1}{2}$ pints) of water. Bring to the boil, cover and then simmer on a low heat for about 20 minutes.

2 Allow the liquid to cool and strain into another pan, pressing the herbs with a spoon to extract all the goodness. Return the strained liquid to the heat and simmer gently until it has reduced to 200 ml (7 fl oz) – you now have a 'decoction'.

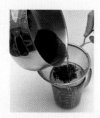

3 Add 450 g (1 lb) of sugar or honey to the pan, and simmer for a few minutes, stirring all of the time until the liquid has the consistency of syrup – don't let the mixture overheat. Take off the heat, allow the syrup to cool and store it in clean bottles.

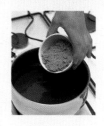

Dosage: one teaspoon three to six times daily for children; two teaspoons three to six times daily for adults.

PREPARING AN INHALATION

Inhaling the smoke from herbs is particularly useful in combating the tightness of the chest and wheeziness that comes with hayfever, but honey must be added to the herb to counteract any rawness and dryness in the throat.

1 Mix one teaspoon of honey with four teaspoons of water. Rub 15 g ($\frac{1}{2}$ oz) of sage together with two teaspoons of any 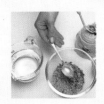 other herb and add the mixture to the honey and water a tablespoon at a time. Rub well into the leaves until they are slightly damp

2 Lay out the herbs on a shallow dish and leave for a few days, so that the water can evaporate, turning from time to time. When the mixture is dry, but not bone dry, place in an airtight tin, label and date.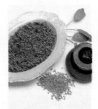

3 Place some of the mixture on a charcoal block, light it and inhale the smoke by standing over it or by using a tube of paper.

The inhalation of smoke from burning herbs, whether rolled as cigarettes, in pipes or, as here on a charcoal block is an ancient practice. Sage is often used as a base herb because it burns well. When mixed with honey and some other herb, such as rosemary, thyme or tarragon, it provides a pleasant and soothing inhalation that can relieve some of the soreness and stuffiness of hayfever.

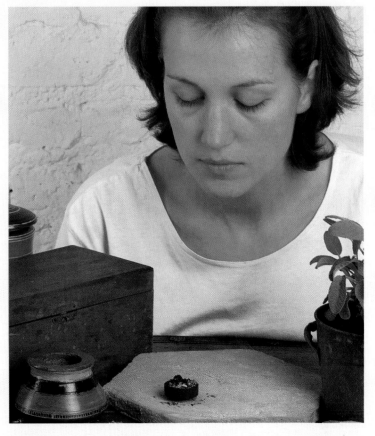

The herbal ingredients to use

All of these ingredients play a part in reducing the symptoms of hayfever, whether singly or in combination. Experiment to find which ones work best for you.

Calendula officinalis (marigold)

An anti-inflammatory and supporter of the immune system, marigold is best taken in tea.

Cinnamomum zeylanicum (cinnamon)

Not only an excellent remedy for colds, which share many of the symptoms of hayfever, cinnamon helps to strengthen and energise the tissues in general. Take as a tea, tincture or inhalation (see pages 50-53), or simply chew a stick of cinnamon for instant relief.

Citrus limonum (lemon)

Together with honey, lemon is a traditional remedy for colds, and so relieves hayfever symptoms.

Glycyrrhiza glabra (liquorice root)

An anti-inflammatory, liquorice helps to protect and heal the mucus membranes affected by hayfever. Chew a piece, or take as a tincture.

Matricaria recutita (chamomile)

An anti-inflammatory and anti-allergic herb, chamomile is best taken as a tea or an inhalation (see pages 50- 53). Chamomile tea is available in teabags from many health-food stores, and inhaling its vapour is especially effective.

Mentha piperita (peppermint)

A decongestant, peppermint can either be taken as tea or inhaled. Try it with chamomile in a tea to clear a blocked nose.

Sida cordifolia

The stem and roots of this plant contain adrenaline, the body's own anti-histamine. Take in a tea, but use sparingly, because too much adrenaline over-stimulates the body.

Thymus vulgaris (thyme)

Taken as a syrup, thyme combats wheeziness and coughs. It can also be used in inhalations.

Urtica dioica (nettle)

A folk remedy for asthma and a general tonic; it makes a delicious tea and can be eaten as a vegetable – cook it in the same way as spinach.

Verbascum thapsus (mullein leaf)

A traditional remedy for bronchitis and dry coughs, mullein leaf is an expectorant, a decongestant and an anti-inflammatory; take as a tea or a tincture (see pages 50-53).

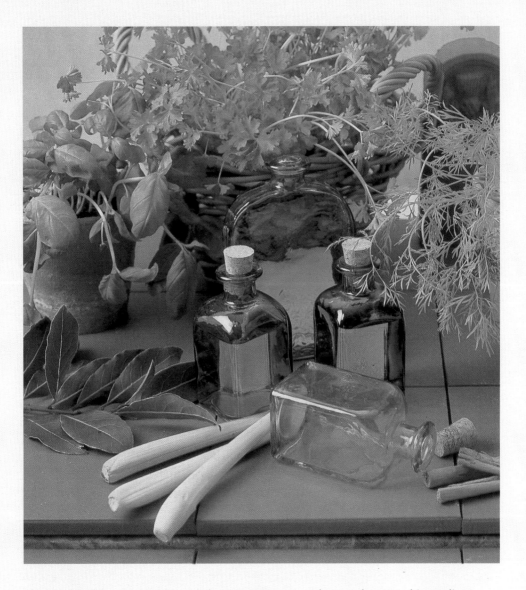

Herbal remedies are simple and cheap to prepare and use only natural ingredients.

Zingiber officinale (ginger)

This warms and loosens up mucus. Chew ginger to unblock sinuses, or take in tea or a tincture (see pages 50-53). It also relieves digestive problems and heartburn.

Honey

Although not a herb, honey has been included here because it is soothing, energizing and healing, and a vital ingredient of herb teas and tinctures (see pages 50-53).

Bach Flower Remedies

The idea that flowers have the power to alter emotional states has been around for a long time – the indigenous populations of America and Australia used flowers as part of their armoury of herbal remedies. But it was not until the 1920s that Dr. Edward Bach (pronounced 'Batch'), a Harley Street pathologist and bacteriologist, devised the system that takes his name.

Bach believed that many of his patients suffered from negative emotional states and that these either caused or aggravated the physical symptoms of which they complained. Becoming disenchanted with the conventional medicine of the day, which tended to treat symptoms rather than the cause of a disease, he retired to a cottage in Wales to search for a new system of healing that would significantly alter negative emotional states.

Bach found that the dew of certain flowers affected his own feelings, and he experimented further by creating a negative emotional state within his own mind and then testing the dew from various flowers to see which ones had a positive effect on his psyche. The outcome was the system of flower remedies that bears his name, comprising remedies for 38 distinct emotional states.

Bach believed that his remedies worked in two ways: they stimulate the body's own healing powers; and they encourage one to combat a negative emotional state in a positive way. As far as hayfever is concerned, they can help keep the psyche on an even keel, calm and well-balanced, and so create the ideal psychological conditions in which the immune system can work to its full potential. And one in particular – the Rescue Remedy – may be useful during a sudden attack of hayfever.

THE REMEDY FOR YOU

Bach Flower Remedies can be bought from most health food shops in concentrated form. Either take them undiluted by placing four drops on your tongue, or dilute them by putting a few drops into a glass of water or fruit juice. Bach Flower Remedies are harmless, so experiment to find which one is appropriate to your state of mind. Try the Rescue Remedy to ease the tension and misery of hayfever – it's a mixture of clematis, cherry plum, impatiens, rock rose and star of Bethlehem. This is one of the most popular of the remedies and is used to combat shock following an accident or to reduce stress. Otherwise choose from the selection opposite according to which of these feelings match your own.

MATCH YOUR STATE OF MIND TO THE APPROPRIATE REMEDY

Impatiens (busy Lizzie)
You are tense, have headaches and are bad-tempered.

Larix (larch)
You expect the worst and lack in self-esteem.

Malus sylvestris (crab apple)
For when things seem to be going out of proportion and you feel slightly unclean.

Olea (olive)
You feel physically and mentally exhausted.

Salix (willow)
You are resentful and bitter about the unfairness of life and feel that the world is conspiring against you.

Ulex europaeus (gorse)
Everything is becoming too much and it seems pointless to try.

Bach Flower Remedies are safe for any condition and can be used by people of all ages.

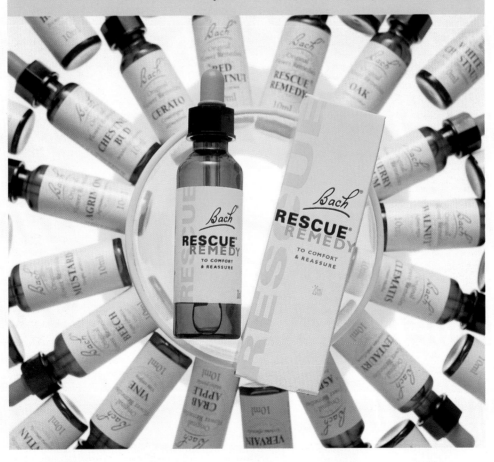

Massage & aromatherapy

Massage has a long tradition as a healing therapy and has been used throughout the world for centuries to treat a wide range of disorders and alleviate their symptoms. A truly complementary therapy, massage can help relaxation and improve the quality of rest, and so allow the body's own healing powers to focus on the medical challenges, such as hayfever, that it faces, rather than the problems caused by stress.

Both head and face massages and back and neck massages are effective in achieving this relaxation in the case of hayfever. Tense, tight upper back and neck muscles, which are often the result of poor posture, can cause headaches, contribute to insomnia and indicate a corresponding over-relaxation in their opposing muscles in the chest – this constricts the airways, which adds to the misery of a hayfever sufferer. A face and head massage – apart from being relaxing – aids the absorption of excess fluids from around the nose and eyes, as well as lessening the tightness and irritability of the facial tissues.

The deep relaxation produced by massage also dissipates the harmful effects of stress (see pages 32-33) and gives the autonomic system a chance to achieve equilibrium, so that the parasympathetic nervous system does not over-react to the presence of allergens and trigger any copious production of mucus and fluids. In addition, a good massage can induce a sense of emotional as well as physical well-being.

PREPARATION

Choose a warm, peaceful room and set aside at least half-an-hour for your massage, making sure that there will be no distractions – take your telephone off the hook or switch on your ansamachine. Undress from the waist up and remove any necklaces or earrings, then lie on a firm surface – either a bed or the floor – with a pillow covered in a warm towel under your head in the case of a head and face massage, or under your lower legs for a back massage. Ask whoever is to give you the massage to wear loose, comfortable clothes and ensure that they have warm hands, short nails and a bottle of massage oil or a mixture of massage oil and aromatherapy oil (see pages 62-63) at hand. Then show them these instructions!

BACK AND NECK MASSAGE

Cover your hands with oil and place them on the body of the person to be massaged – your thumbs should be on either side of the spine below the shoulder blades, and your fingers should point up towards the neck.

1. Stroke firmly up to the top of the neck, across the shoulders and down the back, moulding your hands to the shape of the body. Repeat until the whole area is covered in the oil. Alter the stroke slightly by making circles as you move up the back. Repeat these stroking movements until he or she is relaxed and used to your hands.

2. Starting at the spine at the top of the shoulder blades, use your thumbs to knead the muscles that run up the side of the spine right up to the base of the skull – use small circular movements. (Do not push too firmly at the base of the skull as this can be dangerous). Then stroke down again.

3. Taking one side at a time, knead the shoulder muscle from the neck down to the tip of the shoulder. Use both hands and pick the muscle up in your hands. With one hand, squeeze the muscle without pinching; then relax and squeeze with the other hand. This large muscle can hold a great deal of tension and there may be areas that are tender: if so, use your thumbs to push down on the tender spots, rotate slightly without moving off the spot, hold for a few seconds and release. Repeat five times and then move on to another painful spot or continue kneading. Finish the massage with the same stroking movements as at the start.

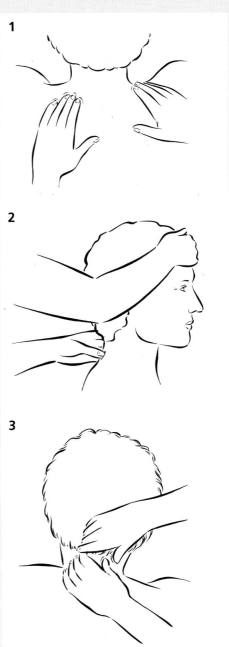

HEAD AND FACE MASSAGE

Lie the person to be massaged on his or her back with the head on a pillow covered with a towel. Stand or kneel behind the head and cover your hands with massage oil (do not allow any oil to go near the eyes).

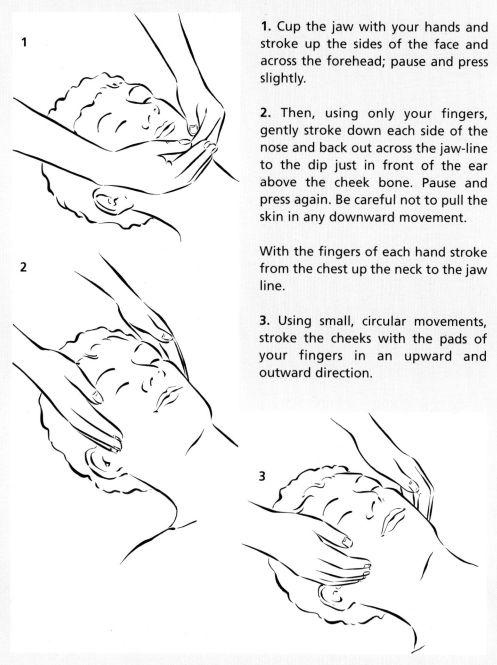

1. Cup the jaw with your hands and stroke up the sides of the face and across the forehead; pause and press slightly.

2. Then, using only your fingers, gently stroke down each side of the nose and back out across the jaw-line to the dip just in front of the ear above the cheek bone. Pause and press again. Be careful not to pull the skin in any downward movement.

With the fingers of each hand stroke from the chest up the neck to the jaw line.

3. Using small, circular movements, stroke the cheeks with the pads of your fingers in an upward and outward direction.

4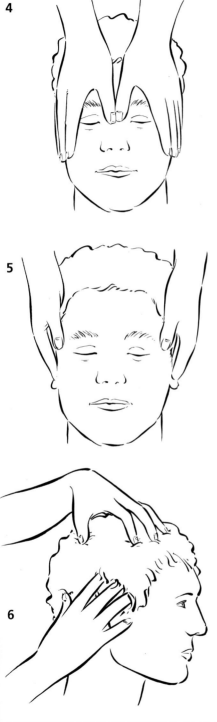

4. Place your thumbs at the bridge of the nose and stroke out to the temples. Pause at the hairline and press. Repeat, moving slightly up the forehead each time until you reach the hairline.

5. Continue the stroking movement, but use either your thumbs or fingers in small, circular movements.

6. Use the pads of your fingers to rub the scalp in circular movements – as though washing the hair thoroughly. You can use scalp oil at this stage, but this will mean that the person being massaged will have to wash his or her hair later.

7. Finish the massage by stroking from the jaw line up to the forehead with your whole hand, pausing over the eyes.

5

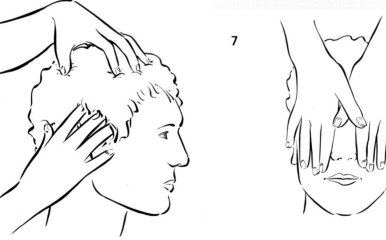

6

7

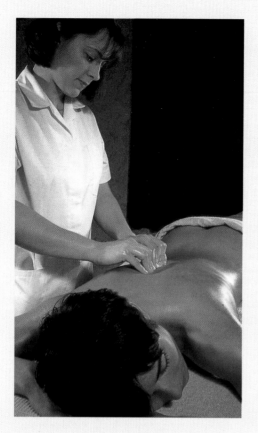

The therapeutic benefits of plant aromas combine well with those of massage.

USING AROMATHERAPY OILS

Aromatic plants have been used for centuries to perfume people and rooms and to camouflage unpleasant smells. But over the years, healers found that the aromas given off by various plants all have different effects on the psyche – smell is analysed in the same area of the brain as emotions – and they have unique therapeutic properties as well.

Aromatherapy is a healing technique that utilises these wonderfully therapeutic properties: essential oils are harvested from the appropriate flowers, herbs and trees, and used in a variety of ways.

Most health stores stock aromatherapy oils. Use a few drops in your bath and inhale the vapours, make an inhalation (see pages 90-91) or mix with massage oil, using two drops of aromatherapy oil to 5 ml of massage oil (in the case of a head and face massage, use only one drop to 5 ml of massage oil and make sure that the resulting mixture is kept well clear of eyes, nostrils and mouth).

Alternatively, mix a few drops with a glass of water in an atomiser, and spray the mixture round the room to freshen the air and to help resistance against minor infections. Make a new mixture each time, as stored aromatherapy massage oil goes off fairly quickly.

Essential oils for hayfever

Boswellia thurifera
(frankincense)
A deep woody fragrance that lingers with calming and relaxing properties. Make up a massage oil and rub into the chest to relieve congestion, or use in the bath as a stress-reliever – it's a wonderful tonic for ageing skin, too.

Cedrus libani
(cedarwood)
A tangy, fragrant oil that helps relive mucus congestion and sinusitis when used in a bath; again, it can also be used as a steam inhalation.

Cymbopogon nardus
(citronella)
A zesty, refreshing oil that helps relieve hayfever symptoms when used in a steam inhaler. It can also be used as a massage oil on the abdomen to clear up digestive upsets.

Eucalyptus globulus
(eucalyptus)
A fresh, tangy fragrance that works fast but dissipates quickly; it has antiseptic qualities and is very refreshing. Derived from the leaves and twigs of the 'Fever Tree', eucalyptus helps relieve hayfever symptoms when used in a bath or as a steam inhalation and works well as a decongestant when used as a massage oil. Try sprinkling one drop on your pillow to help you breathe easily during the night.

Illicum anisatum
(aniseed)
Make up a massage oil and rub into the chest and back to loosen up mucus and relieve sinusitis and other symptoms of hayfever. It can also be taken in a steam inhalation (see pages 90-91).

Matricaria recutita
(chamomile)
A fruity, crab-apple smell with a mellow middle note that is calming and soothes the nervous system. Avoid this, though, if you are allergic to ragweed pollen, because there is a risk of a cross-reaction (see pages 20-21).

Rosa
(rose)
A rich sweet smell that lingers and has anti-inflammatory and mildly sedative properties; try it in the bath to aid relaxation and improve breathing.

Thymus vulgaris
(thyme)
This herb is all-powerful in the fight against infection, but it's an especially useful essential oil when it comes to relieving congestion and easing breathing difficulties. Apply to the chest and back in a massage oil, or use in a steam inhaler.

Acupuncture

In 1973, the Royal Society for Medicine in Britain published a survey of 642 cases treated by acupuncture, covering a variety of disorders. Overall, 37 per cent of patients were classified as 'cured or much improved' following acupuncture treatment. Most importantly, four out of five hayfever sufferers found that their condition had improved after treatment. It was this survey that led to what is now a widespread acceptance by the medical profession of acupuncture as a viable alternative treatment for some medical conditions, including hayfever.

The traditional Chinese belief in acupuncture rests on the idea that the body's life energy – *chi* – is carried through the body, to and from vital organs, along a series of pathways called meridians. A skilled acupuncturist can adjust the flow of energy at the sites where these meridians are closest to the skin, known as acupoints, in order to maintain or restore the balance of energy.

There is no proof – as far as scientists in the West are concerned, at least – that these meridians exist, but several surprising facts about acupoints are now known. First, many acupoints are located where nerves emerge from the deep tissues towards the skin; second, 71 per cent of acupoints correspond to 'trigger points' – areas on the skin that become tender in certain diseases, such as the pain that is felt in the shoulder as a result of liver disease.

There are a number of theories about why acupuncture works, too. One theory is that acupuncture blocks the transmission of pain signals at the spinal cord – but this does not explain how it is effective in the treatment of conditions such as hayfever and arthritis. Another theory is that acupuncture helps to stimulate the production of endorphins, the body's natural painkillers.

However, faced with the statistic that four out five hayfever sufferers can be helped by acupuncture, it probably doesn't matter why or how the technique works. Instead, you should perhaps visit a registered acupuncturist (see pages 124-126) and see for yourself. Be realistic, though: acupuncture is ineffective on around one in four people, as acupuncturists themselves admit,

VISITING AN ACUPUNCTURIST

Before starting treatment, an acupuncturist will diagnose your condition and learn about it in detail by taking your pulse. The adherents of traditional Chinese acupuncture

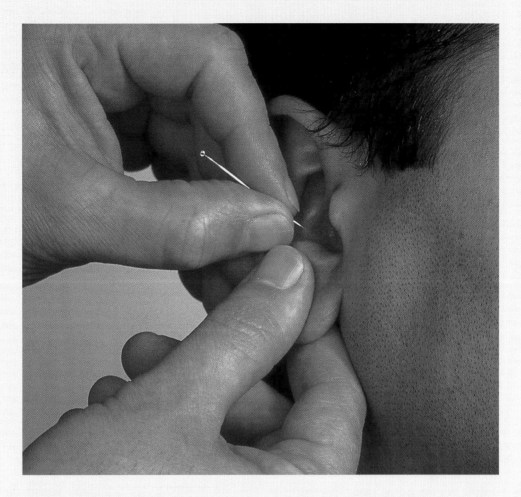

techniques regard this as a vital part of acupuncture: the *Nei Ching*, the first textbook of acupuncture, compiled between 479 and 300BC, describes the 12 pulses – six in each wrist – that must be examined. Each one could have a variety of qualities: 'smooth as a flowing stream', for example, or 'light as flicking the skin with a plume', and these represent various symptoms.

Once the diagnosis has been made, the acupuncturist will insert needles – they are made of silver alloy or stainless steel – with great precision

Acupuncture applied to the ear is known as auricular therapy; it is often effective in treating respiratory complaints.

into any of the 365 acupoints in the body (600 according to one school of acupuncture) in order to adjust the balance of energy that flows along the meridians. The needles are round-tipped, with the result that they divide the flesh rather than pierce it, so there is rarely any blood. Then the needles are manipulated by means of delicate twirling actions or they are pumped gently.

Acupressure

The same basic principle as the one that lies behind acupuncture (see pages 64-65) underwrites acupressure: the aim is to restore the flow of healing energy – *chi* – along special pathways in the body, called meridians. In fact, acupressure is acupuncture without the needles. For this reason, it is an ideal self-help treatment, although you will need a partner to work on some of the pressure points.

Acupressure points are not hard to find, since they are often marked by a slight indentation in the skin and they are often slightly more sensitive than the surrounding area. The illustrations on the next two pages show which pressure points are particularly suitable for the treatment of hayfever symptoms. Measurements are given in finger-widths – make sure, though, that you use your own fingers, rather than

those of a partner, to take the measurements. However, these are not the only points that may be effective, because everyone has their personal 'tender spots', known as *ah shi*. These are often found around the head, neck and face – so experiment.

ACUPRESSURE TECHNIQUES
The rule with acupressure is 'a little and often': around five times a day, for about 15 minutes a session is about right.

1. Use the heel of your hand and the ball of your thumb, taking care not to press down with your fingernails. Aim

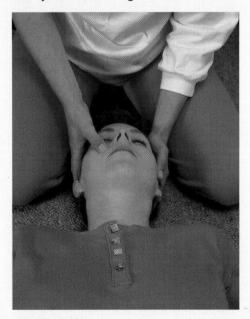

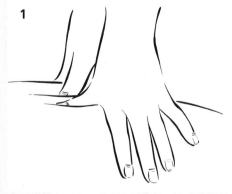

to keep the pressure steady and even, increasing it gradually to a weight of about 5 g – use some kitchen scales to estimate this. Hold for about 20 seconds, then release slowly and gently; wait for about ten seconds, then repeat up to five times.

2. If your thumbs are becoming tired, place your first finger on top of your middle finger – flattening it so that the nails do not touch the skin – and press with this instead.

2

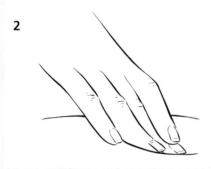

3. Once you have mastered the technique, try making small circular movements, working clockwise, as you apply the pressure.

3

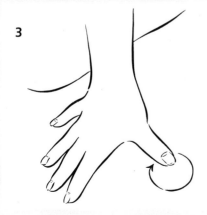

Acupressure points for relief of hayfever

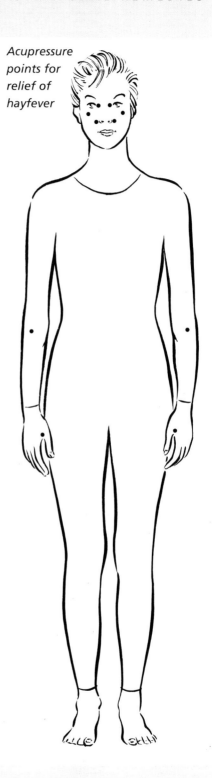

FOR SINUS SYMPTOMS
(and tired eyes)

Apply pressure to pressure point A (see diagram below). This is located just in front of the tear duct, on either side of the nose.

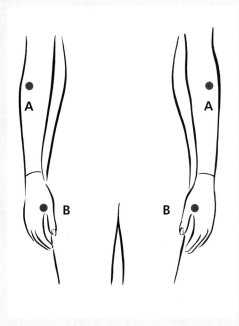

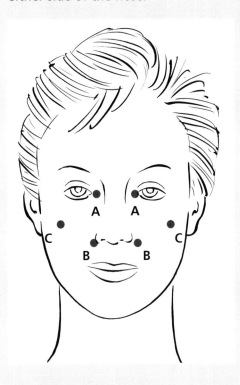

FOR NASAL CONGESTION AND SINUS SYMPTOMS
(and toothache)

Apply pressure to pressure point B (see diagram above). This is located where the base of the nostril joins the face in the small groove on either side of the nose.

FOR COLD SYMPTOMS

Apply pressure to pressure point C (see diagram above). This is located on the point of the cheekbone, on either side of the face.

FOR COLD SYMPTOMS
(and general well-being)

Measure three finger widths below the crease of the elbow and slightly to the outside of the centre line.

Apply pressure to pressure point A (see diagram above). This is located on the muscle of the inner forearm, three finger widths below the crease of the elbow and slightly to the outside of the centre line.

FOR COLD SYMPTOMS
(and pain in general)

Apply pressure to pressure point B (see diagram above).This is located in the webbing between the finger and the thumb on the front of the hand, at the point where the thumb joins the finger.

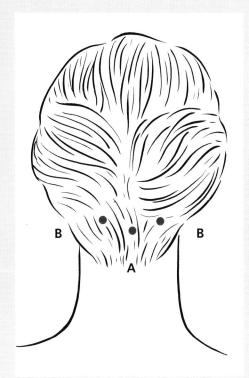

FOR SINUS AND COLD SYMPTOMS
(and headaches, stiff necks and nosebleeds)

Apply pressure to pressure point A (see diagram right). This is located in the mid-line, in the indentation at the base of the skull at the top of the neck. Press up gently, as if into the skull.

FOR SINUS AND COLD SYMPTOMS
(and headaches)

Apply pressure to pressure point B (see diagram above). This is located just to the right and slightly higher than A on either side of the base of the skull. Feel for the indentation on each side of the mid-line, and push gently up and in.

ACUPRESSURE AND SHIATSU

Acupressure should not be confused with shiatsu, although this term means 'finger pressure'. Shiatsu is a Japanese technique that developed separately after ancient Chinese massage techniques had been exported to Japan. It mixes acupressure with a form of physiotherapy with osteopathy and exercise regimes, and should be undertaken by a specialist practitioner. It is not a self-help technique.

Reflexology

Also called zone therapy and reflex zone therapy, reflexology is a healing system that works on the principle that the body's vital energy – *chi* – flows through ten vertical channels down the body, and that the flow is blocked or disturbed during illness. The channels end at the hands, ears and feet, but reflexologists concentrate on the feet because the points on which they work are nearer to the skin, and the feet also provide a larger area on which to work. And because the feet are termination points for the energy channels, they form a map of areas and organs of the body: each channel termination represents the parts of the body through which the channel passes.

By stimulating one of a number of precise points, reflexologists free the energy channel in which they are contained and so treat any tissue or organ through which the channel passes. At the same time, any point on the foot that is a little tender to the touch represents a problem elsewhere in the body, either latent or apparent – which means that reflexology is a preventive as well as remedial therapy.

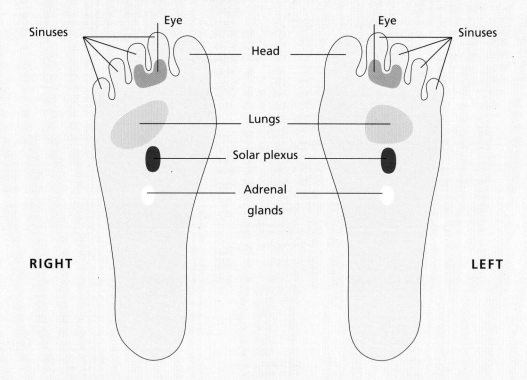

Sinuses   Eye   Eye   Sinuses

Head

Lungs

Solar plexus

Adrenal glands

RIGHT

LEFT

There is no scientific proof that reflexology works in theory, but, nevertheless, it does appear to be successful in the treatment of a number of conditions in practice – often in combination with other complimentary techniques, such as osteopathy, acupressure, homeopathy and naturopathy. To gain the full benefit of reflexology, it is best to consult an experienced reflexologist. Unfortunately, no qualifications are needed to set up in practice as a reflexologist, so it is a sensible idea to consult a national organisation to see if it can recommend an experienced practitioner in your area (see pages 124-126). Otherwise, try massaging the appropriate areas of your feet yourself (see pages 72-73). In the case of hayfever, these are: the big toe and the other toes; the solar plexus point in the middle of the foot; the point that helps the adrenal glands; and the points for the lungs and chest (see illustration, opposite).

REFLEXOLOGY POINTS

Check for any sensitive points by pressing firmly on different areas of the feet and taking note of any tender areas. Make a map of where these points are and work on them.

Knead the points with your thumb (working on tender points on both feet simultaneously, if you have a helper) – but be careful not to dig your thumbnail into the skin. There are two ways of kneading: try pushing down with the pad of your thumb and at the same time rotating the pressure without moving off the spot for 30 seconds (see below, left); or move your arm backwards and forwards for 30 seconds, so that the pressure from your thumb is rocked from side to side (see below, right). Repeat three times on each point.

For hayfever, concentrate on the points highlighted in the illustration opposite for about 30 minutes in total, every other day.

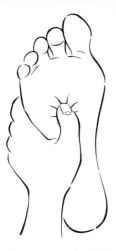

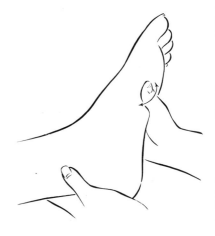

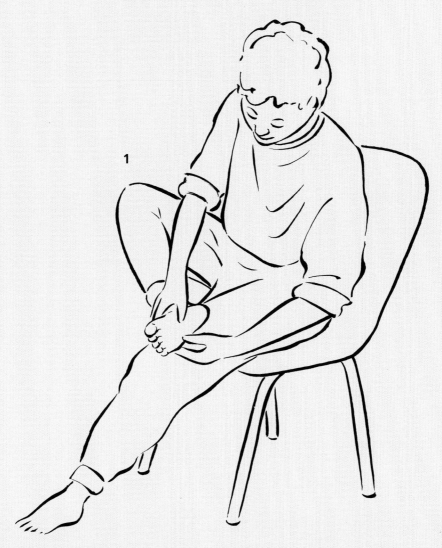

1

REFLEXOLOGY TECHNIQUES

1. Wash your feet thoroughly in warm water and dry them. Sit in a warm peaceful room with one leg crossed over the other – be careful not to strain your back – so that you can reach your foot with your hands; otherwise, ask a partner to help massage you.

2. Massage your foot thoroughly, using an aromatherapy massage oil (see pages 62-63) or talcum powder, stroking and kneading the flesh, especially on the sole of the foot.

3. Move all the joints of the foot, starting with the ankle. Circle the ankle with your hands, moving it first in one direction and then the other; move your foot up and down and in and out.

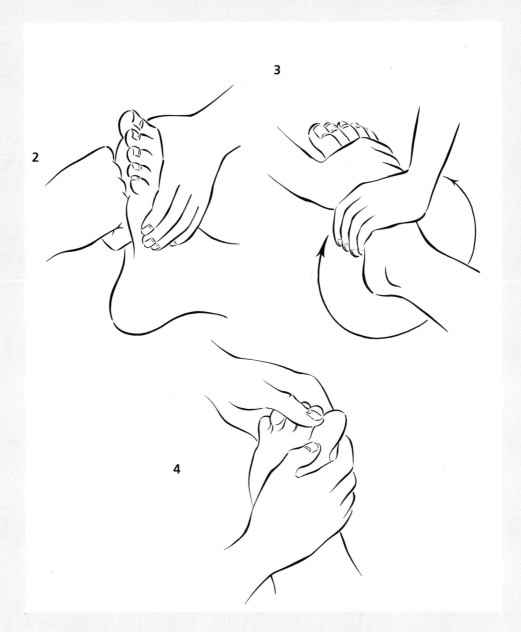

4. Next, take each toe in turn, starting with the big toe, and bend it first backwards and forwards and then from side to side; then finish by pressing on the pad of each toe and gently pulling the toe as though to lengthen it. Finish with a general massage to the whole foot, then repeat the exercise with the other foot.

Once the feet are relaxed, it's time to concentrate on the sensitive reflexology points on the soles of your feet (see illustration, page 70).

Relaxation & exercise

Stress and relaxation are opposite sides of the same coin. We need both to live a rich varied life – in the right circumstances, 'good' stress gives us a wonderful rush of adrenaline, heightened awareness, euphoria and excitement. The trouble is that in modern life there is often a lack of balance between the two sides of the coin: with little 'good' stress and equally little relaxation, harmful stress predominates. Harmful stress is not dissipated; you hold it inside you, worrying about everything, or you carry it around with hunched, tight shoulders as it gnaws away inside you.

As we've seen on pages 32-33 harmful stress affects both your mental and physical state and can aggravate a large number of problems as well as actually causing some of them. Hayfever, in particular, is a case in point, because its mechanism is so closely linked to the stress response. The only way to dissipate the harmful affects of stress is to use up the unspent adrenaline and tension through exercise, or to reduce the amount that is produced by the body by means of relaxation. Exercise and relaxation can not only help reduce the misery of hayfever, but will enhance your general health as well as your physical and emotional well-being.

What exercise you take and the way in which you prefer to relax are a matter of personal taste, and are outside the scope of this book. Nevertheless, it is important that you start some form of exercise – if you are in any doubt about your physical condition, consult a doctor first – and set yourself a relaxation programme (a ten-minute relaxation routine is given on pages 76-77). Many people put off doing so until another day, but that's a mistake – especially as exercise and relaxation can help reduce the misery of hayfever.

THREE STRESS-BUSTING TIPS
Walk tall
Good posture not only makes you appear confident to others, which rubs off on you, but also opens the chest and airways to increase the oxygen intake and reduce mucus levels (see pages 80-83).

Swim
Hayfever sufferers benefit from this excellent form of exercise, and many of them find relief in swimming pools

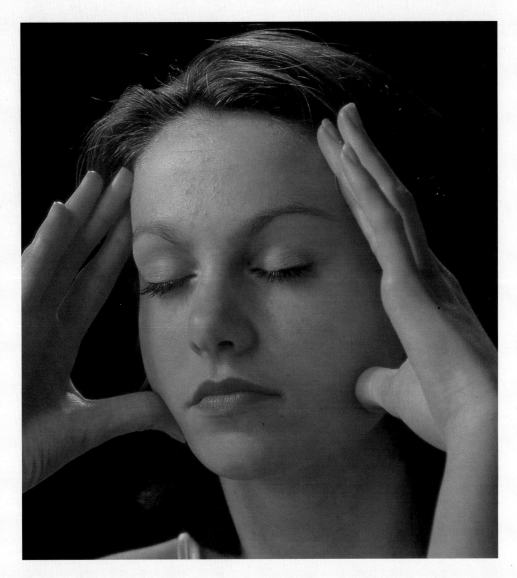

during the pollen season: this is because there is less pollen in a pool, and swimming opens up the chest, especially during the backstroke. And like all forms of exercise, swimming not only uses up the stress hormones but releases endorphins – the body's own painkillers and mood enhancers – and helps the autonomic system to achieve a balance.

Relaxation can help reduce the frequency and severity of hayfever attacks.

Laugh
This is a therapy on its own: the process of laughing releases tension, dissipates excessive fluid around the face and lessens any embarrassment you may feel about itchy eyes or a runny nose.

Ten-minute relaxation

At the very least, you should be able spare ten minutes each day for a relaxation routine – and you'll feel the benefit in all areas of your life, as well as improving your chances of avoiding an attack of hayfever. This simple routine contracts and relaxes each of the main muscle groups in turn to release excess muscular tension. It involves tightening each muscle group and then 'letting go'. Each muscle group may need to be tightened and relaxed several times before it 'lets go' of its tension completely.

This routine is the precursor to many more intensive relaxation routines, but if it is performed properly it is still extremely effective.

Wear loose comfortable clothes and lie down on a mat or a bed in a warm peaceful room where you will not be disturbed – take the telephone off the hook.

1. Place one pillow under your head and another under your knees and rest your hands, either by your side or on your stomach. Then let your mind go blank and take a couple of deep breaths.

2. Start with your toes: crunch them up tightly, hold and then release. Point your foot down and pull up

hard, then release. Circle your ankles in both directions and then crunch up your whole foot and let it go.

3. Move on to your calf muscles, using the same technique, and then up your body to your thigh muscles – you should be able to feel your legs becoming heavier and heavier. If not, tense your whole leg, hold for a few seconds and relax.

4. Move on to your trunk and tighten up your abdominal muscles, your buttocks, your back muscles and your chest muscles in turn – feel the tension oozing out of your body.

5. Next, concentrate on your arms. Start with your fingers and taking each part of your arm in turn up to

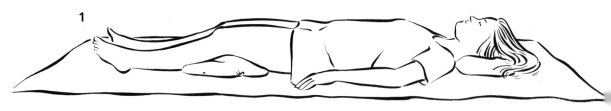

2

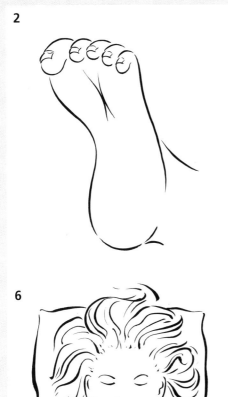

the shoulders – use the same techniques as far as your legs. Feel the warmth spreading throughout your body.

6. Hunch your shoulders up towards your ears and release – it may be necessary to repeat this a few times as we all hold a lot of tension in our shoulders, hayfever sufferers do in particular.

7. The head and neck have been left until last because it is sometimes quite difficult to relax them. Rock your head from side to side, then raise your chin to the ceiling. Grimace to relax your face: frown hard, pout your lips, yawn widely and raise your eyebrows, relaxing between each movement.

8. To finish, tense up your whole body and release, then take a few deep breaths. Now you can either fall asleep, or – even better – do some breathing exercises (see pages 78-79).

6

7

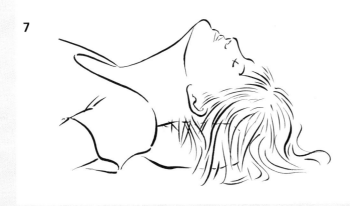

Breathing techniques

Many hayfever sufferers experience breathing difficulties during an attack, and the 30 per cent of them who go on to develop asthma certainly do. During an asthma attack it is vital that you have the ability to control your breathing; during an attack of hayfever the ability to breathe is not affected to such an extent, but it is nevertheless important that you breathe properly, because over-breathing (hyperventilation) can aggravate the symptoms of hayfever or even trigger an asthma attack.

The reason why hyperventilation causes further problems, including hayfever and asthma, is simple: the body needs oxygen for survival. If the supply of oxygen is reduced as a result of a malfunction of the breathing mechanisms – as may be caused by poor air quality, poor posture, a surfeit of mucus or spasm of the chest muscles – the body is put under stress. The muscles contract, the heart races and the blood vessels dilate – all of which achieves nothing, except a sense of panic.

However, correct diaphragmatic breathing increases the supply of oxygen to the body and ensures that carbon dioxide is expelled properly. Practise these breathing techniques so that you can use them in an emergency – they will also stand you in good stead during everyday life.

A BASIC BREATHING TECHNIQUE

To begin, wear loose clothes and lie down on a floor or bed. Place both your hands on the lowest edges of your ribs with your fingers nearly touching.

1. Breathe in deeply and smoothly through your nostrils. Feel your diaphragm as it moves down and out. Your stomach will rise and your ribs will expand upwards and outwards. Hold the breath for a few seconds.

2. Breath out smoothly and evenly, making sure that you empty your

1

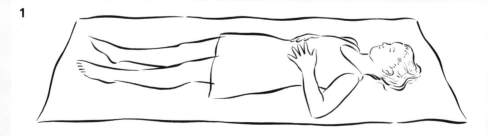

lungs of air. Your ribs will fall down and in and your stomach will sink.
3. Repeat this technique three or four times and, then relax and breath naturally – without thinking about it – for a few minutes. If you breathe too deeply for too long you may feel faint, because too much oxygen may rush to your brain.

SUN AND MOON BREATHING
The basic movements of this technique, which comes from Eastern medicine, are similar to those in the basic technique on the opposite page, but the principle behind them is different. The sun and moon are seen as symbols of the positive and the negative: you inhale positive energy and exhale negative energy.

4. Sit in an upright chair and pinch your nostrils shut with one hand – use your thumb to close one nostril and a finger on the other. Breathe naturally through your mouth as you practise

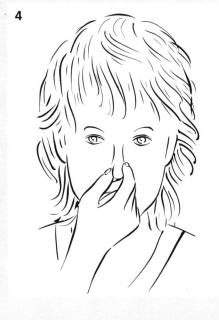

opening and shutting your nostrils by releasing the pressure of your finger and thumb.

When you are confident, inhale deeply through your right nostril (as in the basic technique), keeping the left one shut. Hold this deep breath for the length of time that it took to inhale – this might be difficult at first – and then exhale through your left nostril, keeping the right nostril shut for a similar length of time: the timing ratio should be one part inhaling to one part breath-holding to one part exhaling (represented as the ratio 1:1:1). With much practise, adherents of the technique can achieve a ratio of 1:4:2, but 1:2:2 is sufficient to boost the flow of energy and calm the mind.

After five inhalations breathe through both nostrils, blank your mind and relax fully.

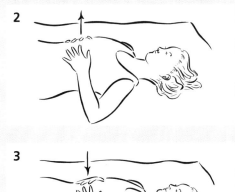

Posture

Good posture is not merely important because it makes you look better, but because it allows the musculo-skeletal system to work efficiently and effectively without tiring. Any deviation in posture, such as rounded shoulders or a flat back, puts strain on the muscles and joints. In the case of a rounded back, for example, the upper back and neck muscles are kept in a high state of tension and the pectoral muscles become too loose, which prevents both groups of muscles from working correctly.

Correct posture is especially important if you suffer from hayfever, because you need as much oxygen as you can get. That means that you must be able to breathe deeply and easily, which, in turn, means that your ribcage must be able to expand to its limit. Rounded shoulders and a head that pokes forward act together to close the airways and prevent the full expansion of the lungs, thus limiting the amount of oxygen available to the body.

The problem is that for every group of muscles there is another group that has an opposing action, and it is the tension between these two groups of muscles that keeps the body in its correct position – the one in which the body's functions, such as breathing, work at maximum efficiency. In the case of rounded shoulders, the 'trapezius' muscle, which runs from either side of the spine to the shoulders from the neck to the mid-back, is in a constant state of contraction, as it attempts to hold the position. That means that the muscles of the chest wall, with which we breathe, are always relaxed, and eventually lose the ability to contract efficiently.

Bad posture can also cause headaches, back problems, foot problems, digestive problems and general tiredness and tension. On the other hand, good posture has a positive effect on the psyche: it reduces emotional stress and tension (see pages 32-33) and helps you to be positive, both about your hayfever and life in general.

THE KEY TO GOOD POSTURE

The position of your head and neck is the key to good posture. If your head is in the correct position the spinal column tends to adopt the correct curves, and the rest of the body follows suit. Therefore it is important that the head is kept in the correct position in relation to the rest of the body – it is all to easy to let the head sag forward when peering up at a computer screen or down at a desk, or while driving.

HOW GOOD IS YOUR POSTURE?

INCORRECT POSTURE

Note rounded shoulders and sagging head.

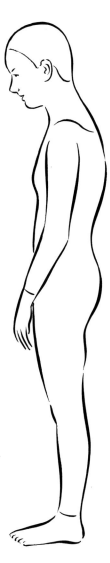

To assess your posture, undress to your underwear, stand in front of a mirror and check the following points. If your posture is not as good as it should be, it might be advisable to learn the Alexander Technique to correct it (see pages 82-83).

The crown of your head should be at the highest point and your ears should be level. Your chin should neither be tucked in nor stuck out, and your eyes should be looking straight ahead.

Your neck should be straight – neither tilted to one side nor the other. Try to elongate your neck at the back by pushing the crown of your head upwards.

Your shoulders should be set back, down and level, but not as rigid as a guardsman on parade.

Your bottom should be tucked in so that your lower back has a small curve, but not so far that you look like a catwalk model.

Your knees should be straight and even but not braced back.

The natural arches of your feet should be obvious, and the weight of your body should be distributed evenly between one foot and the other.

CORRECT POSTURE

Note straight back and neck and level gaze.

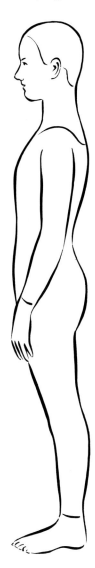

The Alexander Technique

FM Alexander was an Australian actor who found that he often lost his voice during a performance. Doctors failed to solve his problem, so he decided to try to find a solution for himself. Fairly soon he realised that he had a habit of pulling his head down and in when speaking, but he found that if he kept his head level he didn't lose his voice. This observation led him to the discovery that many habits involving bad posture have profound effects on the body – both in mental and physical terms. As a result, he started re-education classes in which people were taught to shed themselves of bad habits and replace them with good ones. Thus, the Alexander Technique was born, and it has since become the best-known posture correction therapy in the West.

The trouble with poor postural habits – whether they involve standing, sitting or walking – is that they feel natural and correct. In fact, any correction of them feels wrong, unnatural and uncomfortable, so that it is all too easy to slip back into the wrong position. For this reason, it is always best to learn the Alexander Technique in classes given by a qualified teacher (see pages 124-126); after you have mastered them you can practise at home to make your postural modifications permanent.

In fact, continual practice is vital – even though an Alexander Technique teacher can move with such fluidity that he or she makes everything look easy. It takes a considerable amount of effort and time to re-educate the mind to accept new positions as normal. You have to become aware of your posture at all times and in all positions, and correct it as and when it slips back into a bad habit. But your movements become freer, easier and more economical as you shed habitual patterns, and this new freedom releases tensions that have been locked into your poor habits. In particular, your patterns of breathing will improve and any inappropriate emotional responses will be reduced.

Some common postural faults that Alexander Technique teachers look for are those of imbalance – whether one arm hangs further out from the body than another or too far in, for example, or whether the knees roll out when sitting and the back is slouched. They also watch to see if there are unnecessary and unbalanced movements during walking, sitting down and standing up. For example, many people poke their heads back and hunch their shoulders while standing up, and then maintain this posture when walking rather than straightening up completely; and too long a walking stride entails bracing the knees with each step, which damages the knee joints and puts the spine out of alignment.

Such observations, followed by the application of the appropriate Alexander Technique to modify the problems, give a wonderful sense of freedom of movement. But they also give rise to greater energy and fuller breathing patterns that both reduce the severity of the symptoms of hayfever and shorten the extent of an attack.

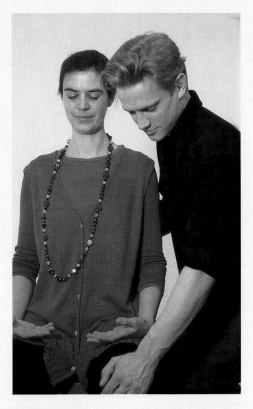

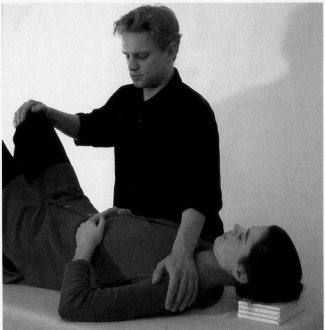

The Alexander Technique is a well-established method of improving posture, with all the benefits that brings. Qualified teachers use their hands to guide their pupils as they perform standard everyday tasks, such as walking, sitting or lying down. Sessions usually last for half an hour or an hour.

Visualisation

We all daydream, and conjuring up pleasant, positive images – winning the lottery, for example – is a pastime enjoyed by all. Visualisation takes this practice a stage further, though, because it puts the ability to daydream, albeit in a focused, concentrated way, to practical therapeutic use. And it has a strikingly successful track record as part of the treatment of many conditions, including hayfever.

It has long been accepted that imagination and suggestion can quite heavily influence the body's autonomic nervous system (see pages 32-33), and this fact is thought to explain why, for example, people can walk on beds of nails: the conscious mind can actually influence the parasympathetic and sympathetic nervous systems to ignore pain signals. In Western cultures we perhaps are more aware of the 'placebo' effect, in which people given a substance that has no therapeutic effect may show signs of improvement if they believe that they are taking a powerful drug.

Visualisation harnesses this power. You are encouraged to concentrate on the detail of your problem and create a mental image of, in the case of hayfever, the mast cells that produce histamine, which causes the symptoms, and focus on the scene as beneficial forces destroy them.

VISUALISING THE BATTLE

Before you start visualising the defeat of the mast cells, relax fully (see pages 76-77) and empty your mind of any extraneous thoughts. Settle in a warm, peaceful room and make sure that you will be undisturbed for at least 15 minutes. Visualisation is a very personal therapy, so choose the images that feel right for you; what follow are merely suggestions. The effect of the therapy can often be enhanced if you teach yourself a gentle form of self-hypnosis (see pages 86-87).

Visualise your face without hayfever symptoms: your eyes are clear and bright; your nose is neither inflamed nor running; your head is clear; and your breathing is even and deep. You are lying on a beach (where there is no pollen) or by a waterfall, feeling relaxed and warm.

MEDICAL ALERT

Do not visualise a field full of grass, a bed of roses or even pollen – cases have been reported of attacks of hayfever being triggered by such visualisations. Concentrate on defeating mast cells instead.

Visualise your nervous system in action: watch the mast cells vanish from your nose; imagine your adrenal glands producing more anti-histamine to fight the histamine and destroy it. Visualise your subconscious deciding that it will ignore pollen or other irritants; tell it that these are harmless to you and should not be fought.

Once you are able to visualise, you will be able to conjure up the picture whenever you need to do so. This ability will help your body fight the over-reaction to allergens and limit the severity of your symptoms.

A 'brain-sync' headset (right) makes use of pulsating patterns of light and sound to make the human mind more susceptible to subliminal self-help messages. Like visualisation (below), it helps the mind to fight hayfever.

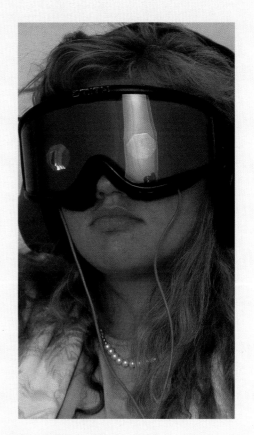

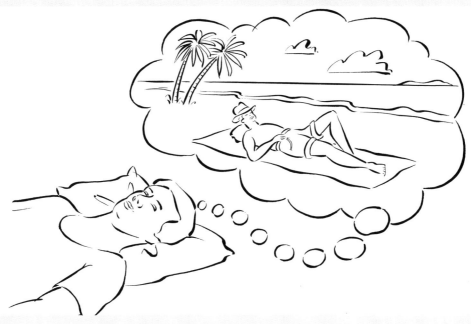

Self-hypnosis & hypnotherapy

You are probably familiar with stage hypnotherapy and the embarrassing things that the hypnotist's subjects are sometimes made to do. But there is a huge difference between stage hypnotism and medical hypnotherapy. The latter is used to induce a trance-like state in which the mind is alert but the body is relaxed, because in this state the mind accepts new ideas readily and subconscious fears and motivations can be changed.

Hypnotism relies on the principle that the while the conscious mind controls and evaluates the world outside and sends orders and messages to the subconscious, the subconscious mind has no logical ability and takes everything it is told as the absolute truth, whether or not this is the case. And once an idea has been planted in the subconscious, it is nearly impossible for the conscious mind to uproot it. For example, if you know that you are allergic to grass pollen you may have the idea – and therefore have planted the concept in your subconscious mind – that an attack of hayfever can be triggered by any pollen, including that from flowers. And even when you know that this is not true (see pages 16-17), you still prefer not to go near flowers

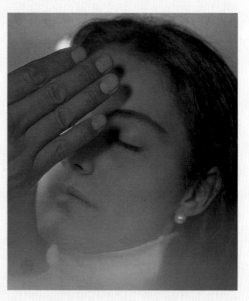

Hypnosis can be useful in resolving any psychological problems affecting allergies.

MEDICAL ALERT

Do not attempt self-hypnotism if you have any history of mental instability; it may be advisable to consult your doctor or a registered hypnotherapy practitioner before any attempt even if you have no such history. In any event, you must ensure that you make the affirmations at each step.

and refuse to have them in the house. However, under light hypnosis this idea can be removed from your subconscious.

Medical hypnotherapy is at its most effective when it comes to relieving stress and helping to resolve a problem that has a psychological component, but it can also increase the positive affects of other healing methods – visualisation, for example. Today, hypnotherapy is one of the most accepted of the complimentary therapies and is used by many conventional doctors. There are reputable organisations and associations in most countries, so contact one of them to find a registered practitioner near to you (see pages 124-126).

SELF-HYPNOSIS

Position an object – anything will do – so that you have to look up slightly to see it. Focus on it, relax completely (see pages 76-77) and let your mind go blank.

Visualise an up and down movement, such as the pendulum of a clock or a see-saw. Watch the movements, breathe deeply and feel yourself becoming even more relaxed.

Count down from ten slowly – try visualising the lights of a lift going down – and as you say each number repeat after it: 'I am sleepy'. By the time you reach the number one you should be in a light, relaxed trance but still completely conscious.

MAKING AFFIRMATIONS IN THE BATTLE AGAINST HAYFEVER

Repeat the following phrases before you say your own affirmations:

'I can wake up completely if there is an emergency'

'I will stay in this trance no longer than thirty minutes'

'I will not slip into a deep trance'

Then make your own affirmations, which must be positive. Try phrases such as:

'I will not be affected by hayfever'

'I will not react to pollen' (or any other allergen)

'My eyes do not itch'

'My nose is not full of mucus'

'I do not have a headache'

'I will sleep well and soundly'

Devise your own affirmations by referring, for example, to the specific causes of your own hayfever.

After you have repeated your affirmations come out of the light trance by counting up from one to ten – by the time you have reached ten you should be fully awake and refreshed.

Hydrotherapy

The healing properties of fresh, clean water have been recognised for centuries, although they are strangely neglected these days – except in Germany, where hydrotherapy is extremely popular, and is accepted as a normal and useful part of medical treatment. In the 19th century, however, people flocked to spas to 'take the waters' for a wide range of mental or physical disorders. Some of the treatments were rather extreme in those days, and when naturopath Vincent Preissnitz opened a spa in Gräfenberg, Austria, his treatments included throwing buckets of freezing water over the patients, rubbing them with wet cloths and making them take ice-cold plunge baths. And they could be dangerous, too: Robert Burns, the Scottish poet, was told to stand up to his armpits in the freezing waters of the Solway Firth for two hours a day to cure his rheumatism – he died a few months later.

Nowadays, however, taking the waters at a health farm or spa is a pleasant, relaxing experience and hydrotherapy is often used by physiotherapists to treat a wide range of problems, from muscular disorders and partial paralysis to hayfever and asthma. Physiotherapists also highly recommend that hayfever sufferers take up swimming, as the air around a swimming pool contains less pollen and other allergens than outside air. This factor helps to make breathing easier, and allows those affected to swim without any shortness of breath. And this is important, because exercise is vital, not only to relieve stress but to ensure that the body's defences are working at maximum efficiency.

Spas and health farms often provide other forms of hydrotherapy, in the form of special baths, for example spa baths or sea-water baths (which are used in a type of treatment called thalassotherapy). A massage is also often available along with the bath.

At home, water can be used to wash away any pollen that has collected on the face or in the hair – and to ease tired muscles, reduce congestion and improve the circulation. In the shower, aim a warm jet of water over your shoulders and your neck, being careful not to choke yourself. Allow the water to massage your face, scalp and shoulders and imagine the mucus draining away with the water.

MEDICAL WATCHPOINT

Do not take a bath with Epsom Salts or a hot and cold bath if you suffer from any circulatory or heart problems.

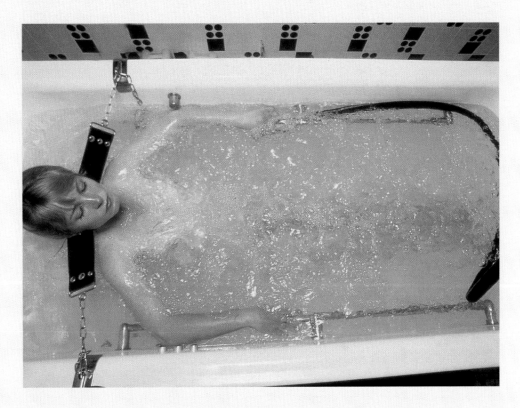

You can do the same thing in a bath, of course, and soak all the tension out of your body by adding aromatherapy oils (see pages 62-63) to the water. Another tip is to add Epsom salts to your bath instead of oils. Also known by their chemical name of magnesium sulphate, Epsom salts neutralise the acid waste products of the body and have a wonderfully calming effect on the nerves. They are available from most health food shops.

There are many different forms of hydrotherapy. Here, a bather is being massaged with pine-scented natural mineral water from 50 or so high-pressure water jets.

HOME HYDROTHERAPY

Put about 1½ kg of Epsom salts into a hot bath – about 40°C (105°F). Lie in the bath for 15 minutes, topping it up with hot water as necessary. You will sweat profusely. Get out of the bath – taking care if you feel faint – and take first a warm and then a cool Epsom salt bath. Then lie down and relax for half-an-hour.

If you haven't got any Epsom salts, try a hot and cold bath, which has a similar effect. Get into a warm bath and then add hot water to heat it up to 42°C (108°F), keeping it at this temperature for five minutes. Then add cold water, cooling the bath down to about 24°C (75°F) and stay in it for five minutes. Repeat three times.

INHALATIONS

We have already spoken about taking herbal preparations in the form of smoke inhalations (see page 53), but the symptoms of hayfever can also be relieved very effectively by the age-old remedy of steam inhalations. These reduce irritation in the membranes lining the nasal passages and sinuses and facilitate the clearing of mucus.

Recently, this remedy has been brought up to date with the introduction of a new inhalation machine called a Virotherm, which can be bought through most pharmacies.

It is quite expensive, but hayfever sufferers find it very helpful. The Virotherm produces a continuous flow of warm, moist air and the manufacturers recommend that you inhale the steam for about 20 minutes at a time.

Even if you don't want to go to the expense of buying a Virotherm there

Steam inhalations are an effective method of clearing congestion and soothing inflamed membranes in the nose and throat, particularly if essential oils, such as eucalyptus or sandalwood, are added.

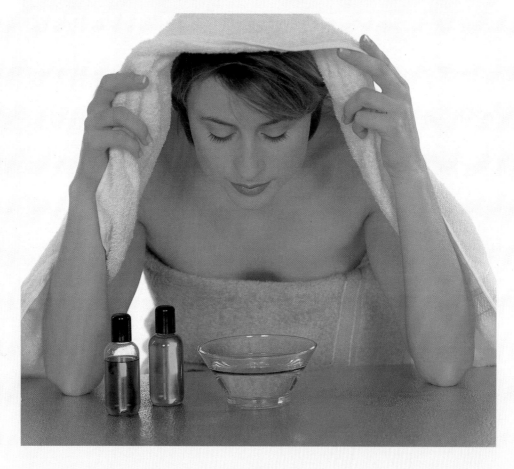

are still a number of the more traditional inhalers and steam kettles on the market – or you can just use a normal kettle. In fact, these old-fashioned devices can be just as effective as the new ones, although not so convenient, and have the advantage that you can add aromatherapy oils to them – pine oil is particularly effective – or other decongestants, such as eucalyptus and menthol. Olbas Oil and Karvol are two well-known herbal remedies that contain these and other ingredients, and you can buy them at most health stores.

HOW TO INHALE STEAM

Boil a kettle of hot water and fill your inhaler – a bowl will do – adding oil or a decongestant if you wish. Bend over the bowl, covering your head, your shoulders and the bowl with a towel, then breathe in the steam through your nose for about 20 minutes; it may help to try the Sun and Moon breathing technique (see pages 78-79) You may need to reheat the water halfway through the process to keep up a good supply of steam.

You can also inhale the steam from an ordinary domestic kettle if you take the lid off so that steam will be produced without the kettle boiling. But it is important that you do not get too close to the kettle as the steam may burn or irritate the sensitive nasal membranes if it is too hot. Make sure, too, that you don't allow the kettle to boil dry or spill any hot water.

After you have finished inhaling, splash your face with cold water and put a cold compress over your nose and sinuses – make one by rolling ice cubes in a tea towel and crushing them with a rolling pin, or simply cover a packet of frozen peas in a towel and apply it to your nose. Leave this on for between five and ten minutes, but no longer. Steam inhalation is a safe technique, and can be repeated as often as you need.

A PINCH OF VITAMIN C

According to recent research in Israel, the mucus formed when you have an attack of hayfever is slightly alkaline while normal mucus is slightly acidic. In the light of this, the researchers placed four drops of a solution created by diluting vitamin C powder, which is slightly acidic, in each of the nostrils of a number of hayfever sufferers. The subjects reported that they felt some relief, so it might well be worth trying the remedy at home. Buy some powdered vitamin C and mix it with water: make the solution very weak to start with – about an eighth of a teaspoon or a pinch of vitamin C to half a pint of water. Boil for five minutes to sterilise, allow to cool and fill a bottle with a dropper – you will be able to buy one from a pharmacist. Administer four drops to each nostril, as required. If the solution stings your nose, you are using too much vitamin C, so add more water.

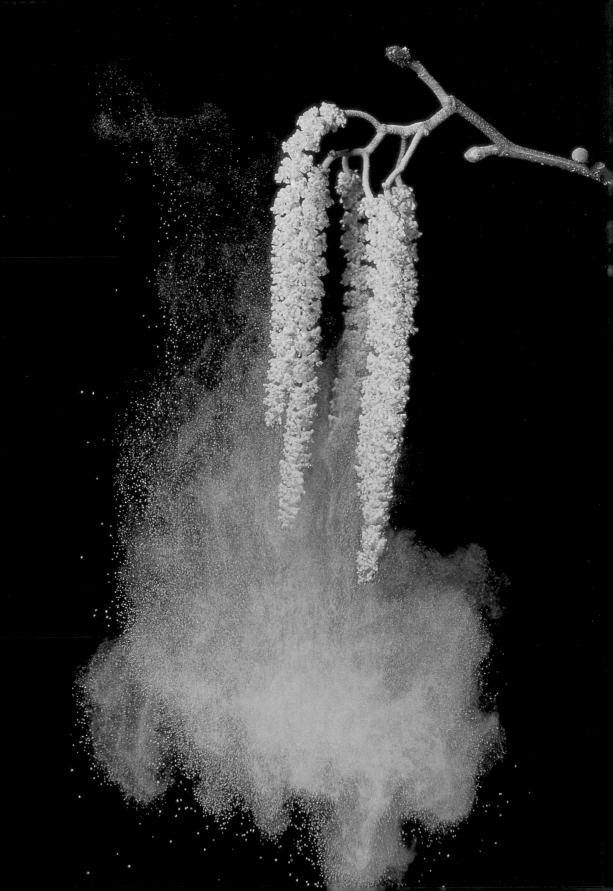

CHAPTER 3

Avoidance & Prevention

Hayfever and other forms of allergic rhinitis are unique, in the sense that they have a specific, identifable cause. However, as we've seen in this book, a substance can trigger an attack when it is related, in a biological sense, to the substance to which you are allergic.

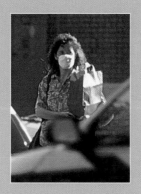

Therefore unlike other illnesses, one form of remedy is to completely avoid the substance responsible or prevent it from coming into contact with you. It's not always easy to do this, in practice since both avoidance and prevention can be both time-consuming and costly. However, even if the avoidance and preventative measures that follow in this chapter do not eliminate your hayfever symptoms completely, they will almost certainly reduce the frequency and severity of attacks and make your life rather more bearable.

KNOW YOUR ENEMY • AVOIDANCE: WEATHER

AVOIDANCE: SPECIAL CIRCUMSTANCES

PREVENTION: IN THE HOME • PREVENTION: OUTSIDE

PREVENTION: IN THE GARDEN • POLLEN AVOIDANCE

USEFUL ADDRESSES • INDEX

Know your enemy

It easy enough to say that you should avoid any substance to which you are allergic and prevent it from coming into contact with you, but how do you know what it is that you have to avoid? The phenomenon of cross-reactions (see pages 20-21) makes it far from easy to find the answer. However, it is possible to devise a structured programme that will enable you to discover what triggers your hayfever, or, at the very least, to give doctors a start when they come to test your reaction to specific allergens.

TAKING YOUR OWN HISTORY

The first thing to do is to buy a notebook, in which you can record everything about your symptoms, when they affect you and what might have triggered them.

Record any family history of allergies – not just to hayfever, but to anything (see pages 30-31), and not forgetting the extended family as well as your mother and father. Record any childhood allergies, not just those that may have caused allergic rhinitis. Next, write down what you can remember of your past attacks of hayfever: how old were you when you first had one?; do you have attacks at particular times or all year round?; does an attack correlate with any particular circumstance?

This information will help you to establish a pattern to your attacks, and it will be invaluable to any doctor who tries to identify the substance to which you are allergic, or confirm your identification of it.

KEEPING A DIARY

The next step is turn your notebook into a diary of your attacks (see opposite page). Each time you suffer from hayfever you should record the following information:

- the time of day
- the day and month
- the outside pollen count – telephone a pollen line to check this (see pages 124-126)
- the weather: the approximate temperature; was it dry, humid, windy or wet?
- a note of the symptoms and how long the attack lasted: how long were your eyes and nose running?; for how long was your nose blocked; was there any wheeziness or tightness in the chest?
- were there any associative factors: had you been in a room with a cat or dog?; had you been outside during harvest-time?; had you been walking near busy traffic?
- what had you been doing in the hour or so before the attack started?

Hayfever Diary

Month:

DAY/DATE	TIME	POLLEN COUNT	WEATHER	SYMPTOMS	POSSIBLE FACTORS	YOUR ACTIVITIES
	6am					
	7am					
	8am					
	9am					
	10am					
	11am					
	12am					
	1pm					
	2pm					
	3pm					
	4pm					
	5pm					
	6pm					
	7pm					
	8pm					
	9pm					
	10pm					
	11pm					
	12pm					
	1am					

Hayfever Diary
Month: *July*

DAY/DATE Monday	TIME	POLLEN COUNT	WEATHER	SYMPTOMS	POSSIBLE FACTORS	YOUR ACTIVITIES
	6am					
	7am	High	Mild/sunny			Cereal + milk
	8am					Caught bus to work
	9am					
	10am					Ate bar of chocolate
	11am					
	12am					
	1pm		Bright sunshine		Lawn being mown	Ate lunch in park
	2pm					Bought bunch of marigolds
	3pm		Humid	Sore eyes, runny nose		
	4pm			Blocked nose		
	5pm			Symptoms disappearing		
	6pm				Heavy traffic	Caught bus home
	7pm			Symptoms returning		
	8pm		Thunder			Pasta for tea
	9pm			Breathing easier		Played with cat. Vacuumed
	10pm			Symptoms returning		
	11pm					
	12pm					
	1am					

It will take several weeks, if not months, before you can start to draw any tentative conclusions from an analysis of this diary – in fact, in some circumstances it may take a whole year for any positive result to actually emerge. Nevertheless, it is worthwhile keeping a diary, because if you take action on the basis of what it reveals, especially if your conclusions are confirmed by a skin test (see pages 98-99), next year might not be so miserable.

READING THE SIGNS

When you have a reasonable amount of data, it's time to see if you can reach any conclusions, and the rest of this section will show you how to test these conclusions in practice. If, for example, your hayfever is mainly confined to the late summer, autumn and early winter, it's likely that your problem is caused by house-dust mites; on the other hand, spring and summer hayfever that persists, though with lesser severity, into the

This diary entry raises the possibility that the allergy is to grass pollen, since the grass was being mown while the person's sandwiches were being eaten; there is also a possibility that there is a cross-reaction with diesel exhaust fumes. However, this diagnosis is only provisional, and many other possibilities need to be ruled out before any definite conclusions can be drawn, so the diary should be kept over a long period. For example, the allergy may not be to grass pollen, but to pollen from some ragweed growing in a flowerbed in the park.

autumn, could well be caused by a pollen allergy that also makes you sensitive to mite droppings. If your hayfever attacks are seasonal, but out of step with pollen counts, you may be allergic to the spores of a particular mould – an allergy can be indicated by a match with the season for that mould and confirmed by a skin test (see pages 98-99).

In the case of pure pollen allergies, however, things are a little simpler, because you can cross-reference the pattern of your symptoms directly to pollen seasons (see pages 114-123): you can then confirm your suspicions by use of avoidance and prevention techniques, and you will know if you are correct if they are successful at reducing the number and severity of hayfever attacks, and you will be able to set a pattern of living for the future.

By the same token, your diary entries may show, for example, that the bout of hayfever you always suffer after visiting your aunt, say, may be associated with the fact that your aunt has a cat, which excerbates your hayfever symptoms.

Even if no firm conclusions spring to mind when you examine your diary, it may be that a specialist can derive useful information from it, so take it to any consultation. A sample diary is shown on page 96, together with an entry form that you can photocopy (see page 95) and stick into your own notebook.

SKIN TESTS

Your diary may well lead you to suspect the identity of the substance to which you are allergic, or at least the family to which it belongs, but confirmation of its precise nature can only come from the results of a skin test. There are four different types of skin test – a scratch test, a prick test, an injection and a patch test – but all rely on the same principle: a series of different allergens are put in contact with the skin tissues to see which one causes an allergic reaction.

Scratch tests and prick tests are the ones most often used by allergists. Both are easy to administer and are no more painful than a pinprick, and

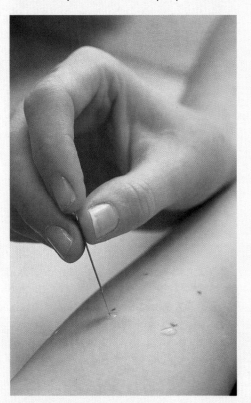

they also have the advantage that as many as 30 different tests can be carried out at the same consultation.

In the case of a scratch test, the skin is scraped with a needle and a sample of a particular allergen is dropped on to the scratch: if the subject is sensitive to that allergen, the area of the scratch will become red and swollen – the larger and redder the bump, the greater the sensitivity.

In prick tests, the allergen is dropped on to the skin and this is then pierced with a needle or lancet in order that the allergen can come into direct contact with the mast cells in the underlying tissues: the response is positive if the site becomes red, swollen and itchy.

On certain occasions, an allergist injects allergens into the superficial layers of the skin about an inch apart. This is the most accurate of the various types of skin test, but is usually only performed if there is a definite suspicion of what the

In a skin-prick test, the commonest form of medical test for the causes of hayfever, small quantities of suspected allergens are injected into the skin of the forearm or back using a small needle or lancet. After 10 or 20 minutes, the skin is inspected for any signs of swelling and inflammation. Where these signs are found, there has been an allergic skin response to that particular allergen. The size and redness of the swelling indicates the strength of the reaction.

allergen might be – this is where your diary comes in handy. A generalised, non-specific reaction to the allergen is ruled out by administering a highly diluted dose first. As with the other tests a redness and soreness indicates that the person is allergic to that particular allergen.

A patch test works on the same principles as the other tests, but in this case the skin is not ruptured at all. The allergen is placed on a piece of soft cloth or paper and stuck on to the skin by a plaster, which stays in place for 48 hours before being removed. Any reaction at the site indicates a sensitivity to the allergen. Patch tests, however, are usually used for skin allergies rather than hayfever.

BLOOD TEST

If a person has a skin infection which prevents them from having one of the skin tests previously described, a blood test can be taken instead.

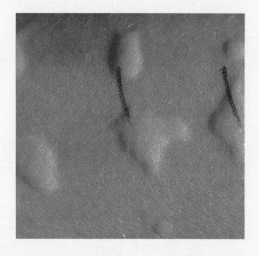

Close up of a patient's arm showing a series of skin reactions to allergenic substances, previously injected or scratched into the arm.

This helps to determine the amount of imunoglobulin E or IgE (see pages 12-15) in the patient's blood. The test is usually carried out for a particular type of IgE, such as IgE to ragweed or grass pollen antigens.

VEGA TESTING

A VEGA test, also known as a vegetative reflex test, measures the concentration of certain compounds within the body. The homeopath takes electronic readings from a rack of tubes which contain homeopathic preparations of naturally occurring bodily substances. The homeopath compares this with a reading from acupuncture points on the patient's foot (see pages 64-65). A reading indicating an excess of any compound in the body is used to indicate the nature of the patient's ailment. A homeopathic remedy may then be prescribed.

MEDICAL ALERT

A positive reaction to an allergen is normally confined to the site of the test, but in rare cases, when the subject is extremely allergic to a substance, the test may trigger more generalised symptoms such as wheezing, general itching, hives and sneezing. In exceptional cases a skin test can trigger an asthma attack or even lead to anaphylactic shock (see pages 28-29). For this reason it is important that you consult a qualified allergist who has resuscitation equipment on hand.

Avoidance: weather

Once you know your enemy, you can start to work out some strategies to avoid it. The first thing to do is to take special precautions during the season for the pollen to which you are allergic – telephone one of the pollen lines to find out when this is (see pages 124-126), or look in a botanical book.

During the months when you are at risk, you should pay particular attention to weather conditions, because it is these that govern what time of the day pollen is most likely to be present in the air.

In general, plants release pollen early in the morning, although some tree pollens, such as birch, are released in the afternoon. Times vary, according to the species – ragweed, for example, tends to release pollen from around dawn to 9am, while grass pollen is released from about 7.30am to 10am (although some grasses release pollen later in the day). If it is damp and cold, the pollen will not leave the flower, and if it is raining, the pollen will be washed away: so you are unlikely to have an attack of hayfever in either case. If it is mild and there is a light breeze however, the pollen will be blown around in the air and a hayfever attack is a possibility.

The trouble is that often things are not that simple. On a warm, sunny day, for example, the morning sun will warm up the air and rise into the atmosphere, taking the pollen with it. The pollen will stay high in the atmosphere until the air cools, either because the sun has set or the weather has changed, but when the air has cooled, the pollen will fall back to the ground. This means that pollen may not begin to fall, and give rise to an attack of hayfever, until a few hours after sunset – or later than this if you live in a city, where the ground air stays warmer for longer.

INVERSION
An added complication is the phenomenon known as 'inversion'. In some geographical circumstances, a layer of cold air hugs the ground, even though there may be warmer air above it. Typically, this happens in a valley or low-lying area surrounded by higher ground. The result is that the air at ground level does not rise, and all the pollen is trapped near the ground, together with any other pollutants that there might be – in a city, the effect would be described as a 'smog'. However, even in the country there may be a build-up of pollen in a valley without any visible smog – if this is the case, you will be in danger of having an attack of hayfever throughout the day, unless it is damp or raining.

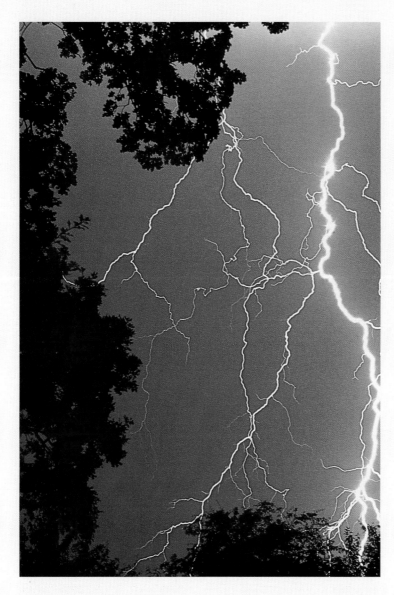

Thunderstorms affect hayfever sufferers in several ways. In the period before a storm, symptoms are likely to be worse. But when the rain comes, the air is washed clean and the likelihood and severity of hayfever attacks is reduced.
Lightening is also good for hayfever because it increases the proportion of negative ions in the air (see pages 108-109).

Keep a close watch on weather conditions, both current and forecast, during the season of pollen to which you are allergic. The main danger comes when a warm, dry day follows a period of cold and dampness, which will have caused a build-up of pollen in the plants. Then – unless inversion is a factor – you should take all possible precautions against exposure to pollen (see pages 102-113) in the late evening if you live in the country, or from the late evening to late at night if you live in a city. But if you live in a valley or low-lying area surrounded by high ground, you may be at risk all day long on any day on which there is no rain or dampness.

Avoidance: special circumstances

There are times when an attack of hayfever is not just unpleasant and debilitating, but can have unfortunate – or even dangerous – consequences on others. At such times, taking the appropriate measures to avoid an attack is not just sensible from a personal point of view, but an obligation.

There are two occasions, in particular, when consideration for others becomes a priority: when you are driving a car, and when you have a baby. And, of course, avoidance on such occasions will help to make your life easier, too.

DRIVING

When you think of roads, you tend to think of tarmac and white lines. You forget the grass verges, hedgerows and lines of trees that border the verge: but these are major sources of pollen. Add to that the fact that you may well be crawling along the road in a traffic jam, and that the very motion of a car stirs up sufficient breeze to make large quantities of pollen airborne, and you have a strong liklihood of a hayfever attack. And having a hayfever attack while driving is not just unpleasant and uncomfortable, but dangerous, too – both to yourself and others: sneezing, watery eyes, a headache and all the distraction that hayfever causes are hardly conducive to safe driving.

The simple answer – though easier said than done – is to keep your windows shut when driving during the hayfever season. Unfortunately, this is likely to coincide with dry, warm weather, and nobody wants to sit, sweltering in their car. But there is a solution, though one that comes at a price. Ideally, you should buy a car that has an air-conditioning system, since these can remove as much as 95 per cent of the pollen in the air. Otherwise, buy one of the special pollen filters that are available. These can be fitted over the air intake – ask your car accessories dealer for advice. In addition, it's also worth fitting an in-car ioniser (see pages 108-109).

PREVENTIVE PARENTHOOD

As we've seen throughout this book, a tendency to allergies, though not to specific allergies, is inherited (see pages 30-31). This does not mean that your child will necessarily develop an allergy – or hayfever, in particular – even if both you and your partner suffer from allergies, because there are measures you can take, as a parent, that can reduce the likelihood that this will happen.

The most important time, when it comes to reducing the chances that your child will suffer from hayfever or any other allergy, is the first year of his or her life, starting from birth. There are two reasons for this: first, exposure to potential allergens during this time seems to predispose (in those with an inherited tendency) to developing an allergy later in life; second, breastfeeding is thought – though there is some argument about this – to help prevent an allergy from developing.

Whether there is a convincing argument or not, it makes sense to err on the side of caution. First, you should breastfeed your baby right from the start, if possible – and that means making sure that no supplemental bottle feeds are given as a matter of routine (as they are in many hospitals), since these may sensitise your baby to cow's milk. Second, you should ensure that your baby is exposed to the minimum quantities of potential allergens during the first year of his or her life. That means that you should not buy a new dog or cat to keep the baby company – it might even be sensible to keep an existing pet outside the house; and that you should not move house or spring clean just before your baby is due – because you run the risk of stirring up house-dust and the mites it contains.

PETS

The problem of what to do with an existing pet, especially a dog, is a difficult one for many families. It can seem particularly hard to cast a faithful family friend out into a kennel when they are used to the comfort of a warm fireside, and to banish them from the room whenever the child is around. Sometimes it is simply impractical to do so. In these cases, it may be best to allow the existing situation to continue.

Keep the pet and its surroundings clean – wash dogs regularly since they can also carry pollen into the house – and keep a very close eye on the situation. If your child, as he or she grows, begins to show signs of hayfever in the presence of the pet, then action can still be taken. It may be enough to restrict the pet to one part of the house or a single room. If this fails, then the pet will have to be kept out of doors. Only as a last resort should the pet be found a new home. It may help to give them a new, non-allergenic pet such as a hamster.

PLANNED PARENTHOOD

There may be other ways in which you can reduce the liklihood of your children developing hayfever. There is some evidence that children born at the beginning of the pollen season are more likely to develop hayfever in childhood. Therefore, if possible, it might be a sensible idea to plan the pregnancy in order to avoid having a baby at this time of year.

Prevention: in the home

Commonsense dictates that one of the most effective ways of preventing an attack of hayfever is to make sure that your home, at least, is an allergen-free refuge. That's very much easier said than done, of course, so the next few pages list some practical measures that can make all the difference. Concentrate on the ones that will help remove the particular allergens to which you respond.

The prime cause of hayfever is pollen, so it makes absolute sense to take every possible step to exclude pollen from your home. If you now know the types of pollen to which you are allergic (see pages 94-99), focus your efforts on the appropriate times of year when your pollen is in the atmosphere (see pages 114-123).

EXCLUDING POLLEN

Remember that the pollen count rises at certain times of the day and in certain weather conditions (see pages 100-101), so keep your windows tightly shut during these times in order to minimise the amount of pollen that enters your home.

Bear in mind, too, that pollen rises in warm air, so if you live on the top floor of a high building there will be a high pollen count outside your windows on most dry, warm days. Make the most of any rain to air your home thoroughly, or open your windows in the late evening – you may have to close them again at sunrise, though. Always keep your windows shut and stay inside if anyone is mowing the grass nearby, or during harvest time if you live in the country.

Of course, you have to go outside sometimes, even during the pollen season. One way of avoiding contaminating your home with pollen that has adhered to your clothing is to keep two different sets of clothes: change as soon as you come home and keep your outdoor set in a tightly fitting cupboard, separate from your indoor clothes. (Try to avoid clothes that are made of wool or provide bobbly surfaces to which pollen can cling easily.) Then rinse your hair and face immediately to remove any pollen that may have stuck to your skin – it's worthwhile doing this before you go to bed in the evening, too.

All the above may be good advice, but it is very difficult to follow in practice in most family homes. However, there is a compromise: attempt to keep your bedroom and one other room free of pollen. Grains of pollen are larger than many other allergens, and settle to the ground quite quickly when the air is still, taking about seven minutes in an average house. You can take advantage of this fact by asking a friend who does not suffer from hayfever to sit in your chosen room for at least seven minutes with the door shut and then vacuum the floor and soft furnishings and wet-wash the furniture. Your friend must then creep out of the room, making sure that he or she doesn't slam the door and create movement in the air. Your room will then be relatively clear of pollen, and likely to stay so, unless you abandon your other precautions or move around energetically.

When it comes to your bedroom, it's worth putting a cotton cover over your bed and pillows when you get up and rolling it up carefully when you retire for the night, avoiding stirring up any pollen that has settled during the day.

FILTERS

Unfortunately, the presence of children and pets mitigates against this plan, because it is almost impossible to keep the air in your house still when they are around. (Long-haired pets, in particular, can carry large amounts of pollen into a house on their fur, so they should be showered frequently and always be kept out of the bedroom and preferably out of at least one other

room.) If this is the case, the answer may be to buy an air filter in order to sieve the pollen from the air.

A number of different types of filter exist, but the best are HEPA filters (High Efficiency Particulate Air), which must remove 99.9 percent of particles from the air to merit their description. However, it is important that you buy one powerful enough to 'clean' the air in a room the same size as yours four times an hour. Various models are on the market, but it is best to approach a manufacturer who will let you test the device at home before

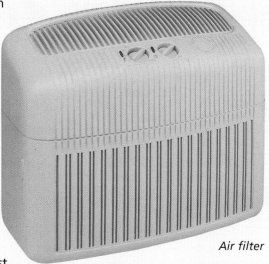

Air filter

you buy it. Otherwise, you may wish to consider installing air conditioning: this is an expensive business and domestic systems are rarely found in Britain, but air conditioners can be very effective at removing pollen and other allergens from the air, and also at keeping the air dry.

MOULD SPORES

Cutting down on the movement of air is a good way of tackling the problem of pollen in the home, but it has annoying side-effect of increasing humidity. And warm, humid, still conditions are ones in which mould thrives (see pages 22-23). The answer is to use a dehumidifier that reduces the moisture from the air to under 45 per cent – some models can reduce moisture even further, but they should not be left on in a room in which someone is sleeping.

MITES

House-dust mites (see pages 24-25) thrive in centrally heated, draught-free houses that have fitted carpets, heavy curtains and soft furnishings, and, like mould, they love humidity; they are also extremely tenacious. Apart from buying a humidifier, the obvious, though rather drastic solution is to throw out all of your carpets and have wooden floors, but if this is not feasible it's well worth considering laying short-pile synthetic carpets.

Hang cotton, washable curtains and wash them frequently at a high temperature (60°C/140°F) – you should fit washable covers on your chairs and sofas as well. Turn down the thermostat on your heating, and if possible leave your bedroom without heating.

Clean and vacuum your house regularly – at least twice a week – concentrating not just on the carpets but also on your bedding, soft furnishings and sofas. It is well worth buying a powerful vacuum that has a special allergen filter – ask the Allergy Foundation (see pages 124-126) for a list of manufacturers and stockists. Mop floors wherever possible, but make sure that they dry quickly.

Furniture should be wet-washed so that as much dust as possible is picked up, and then dried with a cloth to prevent any water marks from developing; try to keep knick-knacks to a minimum or lock them up in a display cabinet. Dry clothes outside, but give them a good shake in the pollen season before bringing them in or use a dryer – never

A powerful vacuum cleaner fitted with a fine filter is essential in the fight against house-dust mites. Models that use a miniature tornado to create a powerful vacuum are much more effective than conventional models.

dry clothes over radiators as this increases the humidity on which dust mites thrive.

One main reservoir of mites in your home is likely to be your bedding and mattress, because it is in bed that you shed much of your dead skin. High temperatures kill the mites, so at the very least it is sensible to choose bedding made from synthetic materials or cotton that can be washed at high temperatures (60°C/140°F or over) – dry cleaning them is not as effective. Wash linen and pillows weekly and duvets and blankets fortnightly. Alternatively,

Bedlinen is particularly attractive to mites and should be washed regularly; the scent of lavender helps to combat sleeplessness.

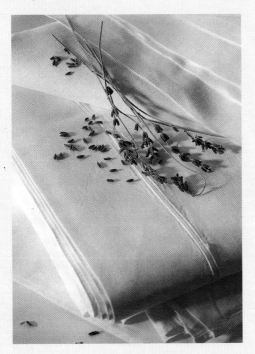

you can buy special dust-free and 'anti-allergy' duvets and covers that are non-toxic to humans but kill mites – contact the Allergy Foundation (see pages 124-126) for addresses of manufacturers and stockists.

If neither of these options is possible, adopt the practice, which is common in continental Europe, of airing your bedding by hanging it out of a window during the day – cold, dry weather is ideal, since the mites cannot survive in cold, dry air. You can also use coldness as a weapon against mites by placing your pillows in a bag and placing them in your freezer overnight; the next day, wash them at a high temperature and follow with two hours in a hot dryer.

All of these precautions will help to keep the population of mites down, but do not go to the root of the problem, which is likely to lie in your mattress. Often the best thing to do is to buy a new mattress and seal it in a plastic cover before use – similar to the ones used on hospital beds or fitted when a child wets its bed. Make sure any seams are air tight, and cover them with packaging tape if necessary.

If funds allow, a better bet is one of the new 'allergen-proof' covers made from a micro-porous material' that allows the mattress to breathe but prevents house-dust mite infestation – these are also less slippery and hot than plastic covers, and are stocked by a variety of pharmacists.

Otherwise, try treating your old mattress with acaricide (mites are more spiders than insects, and this is more effective than an insecticide). However, this treatment should not be undertaken by the person who suffers from hayfever, because there is a risk of a cross-reaction to it (see pages 20-21). (Liquid nitrogen can also be used to kill off the mites, but this must be performed by an outside specialist.) Afterwards, the room and all its contents must be vacuumed thoroughly to remove both the dead mites and their droppings.

IONISERS

So far we have been discussing practical measures to control allergens, all of which take a great deal of time and effort. However, there may be a simpler way: to buy an ioniser. This is certainly something that you should consider because research undertaken at the University of Surrey found that 70 per cent of people using ionisers said that their hayfever symptoms had been significantly helped.

weather conditions – when there is a warm, dry wind, for example. However in cities and towns, pollution, dust and fumes can eliminate the negative ions in the air, and the ratio can fall from one negative ion to three positive ions.

It has been found that a preponderance of positive ions in the air makes people feel irritable and bad-tempered, increases the incidence of general malaise and headaches and worsens symptoms of hayfever and asthma. You will almost certainly have experienced the feeling yourself: before a storm, people often feel lethargic and depressed as negative ions are reduced; after the storm has broken they feel invigorated and cheerful afterwards. This is because negative ions are formed around moving water, such as rainstorms, waterfalls, rivers and the sea.

Ionisers are devices that emit negative ions into the atmosphere, and so freshen the air by increasing the proportion of negative ions to

The principle of ionisation is fairly straightforward. Basically, the air that we breathe contains electrically charged particles that can carry either a positive or a negative charge – these charged particles are known as 'ions'. In the countryside, there is normally a balance between the charges, though there are more positive ions in the air during certain

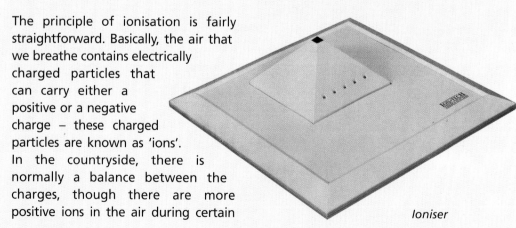

Ioniser

positive ions. They can also attract and remove dust, smoke and pollen particles from the air, and so many of its allergens. There is a physiological reason why they work, too: when the air is rich in allergens and positive ions, the cilia – hair-like filters in the nasal passages – become almost stationary; but negative ions increase their mobility, so that they can move the allergens away from the sensitive nasal passages and prevent an inflammatory reaction (see pages 26-27). Negative ions also have an anti-histamine effect (see pages 12-15), and quite large reductions in blood histamine levels have been found after the use of an ioniser.

Ionisers vary in size: you can buy one that's as small as a transistor radio or, if you work in an open-plan office, as large as a computer. They are widely available and many manufacturers will allow you to have one on a trial basis, so that you can experiment to see which size is right for your room; one solution, though, is to buy a portable ioniser that can be carried from room to room.

Whatever your choice, it is worth trying an ioniser for at least two months because some people find that it only starts to help after this period. However it has to be said that ionisers do not always work – some people find them no help at all.

High levels of pollution fill the air with positive ions, which make hayfever symptoms worse. Rainfall, waterfalls, lightening and the sea are natural ionisers, filling the air with beneficial negative ions.

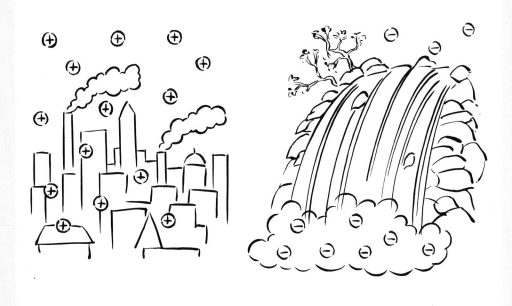

Prevention: outside

Keeping the levels of allergens down inside your house is one thing, but it's impossible to reduce them when you are outside. Avoidance is one answer (see pages 100-103): if at all possible, try not to leave your house or workplace at times when there is a high pollen count or air quality is low.

It is sensible to avoid any substance that may cause a cross-reaction (see pages 20-21), though this can be particularly difficult if you live in a busy town or industrial area. In the latter case you are likely to be exposed to sulphur dioxide particles and acid droplets, which are emitted from factories and power stations; and in the former to exhaust fumes, which cause the levels of nitrogen and ozone to rise. Diesel fumes are a common trigger for cross-reactions, so buy a car that runs on petrol and avoid taxis, lorries and buses, all of which run on diesel – especially during the heavy traffic of the morning or evening rush hour or when air quality is poor.

Of course, there will be times when it is essential for you to leave the house. One solution to the problem is to wear glasses, and many hayfever sufferers routinely wear sunglasses that only darken in the presence of

Face masks filter out pollen and other allergens and can be hugely beneficial for hayfever sufferers.

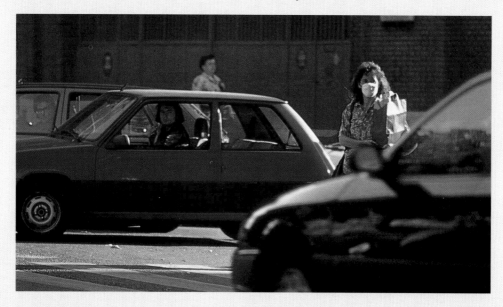

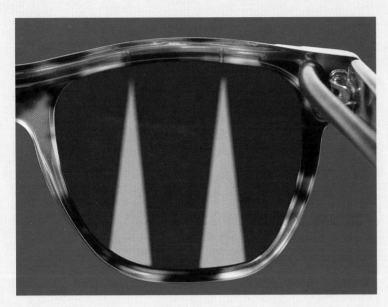

Anti-hayfever spectacles use a cushion of air from a small battery-powered pump to keep pollen from settling on to the eye. The chevrons show the flow of filtered air from two small vents in the frame.

light during the spring and summer. These give some protection, but pollen can get around the side of ordinary glasses easily enough. You could prevent this from happening by wearing a pair of goggles bought from any DIY retailer, but this solution may leave something to be desired in terms of fashion.

A more practical idea is to buy a pair of prescription glasses if you use them, or sunglasses or glasses made of plain glass if not, that have enclosed sides – such glasses can be obtained from most opticians.

WEARING A MASK

Sometimes even wearing enclosed glasses gives insufficient protection and an allergen can cause a hayfever attack by entering your body through your nose and mouth, especially in busy traffic or during harvest time in the country. In such cases the only

thing to do is to wear a mask that covers the nose and mouth as well as wearing glasses.

Three different types of mask are available, and it is important that you choose the correct one. First, there is the 'nuisance dust mask', which can filter out chemical irritants, pollen and other large particles, but not pollen fragments or smaller allergens – these can be bought at most pharmacists and health stores. Ordinary dust masks, which are used by builders and decorators, filter out fine particles, but not chemical irritants such as diesel fumes. They are obtainable from builder's merchants and DIY stores. However, the best type of masks to buy are the ones known as 'dust respirators'. These filter irritants and allergens down to a very small size, but they are expensive. Contact the Allergy Foundation (see pages 124-126) for information on stockists.

Prevention: in the garden

It is difficult to make your garden a pollen-free area because even if you avoid having plants to whose pollen you are allergic, you cannot prevent such pollen being blown into your garden from the gardens of your neighbours. Nevertheless, it is sensible to take as many preventative measures as you can.

Many hayfever sufferers are allergic to grass pollen, of which the lawn is the prime source. The drastic option is to pull up all the turf and lay down paving stones, but if this is not possible, you should make

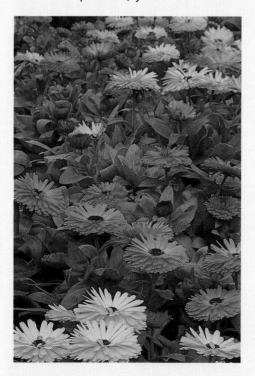

sure that the grass is cut frequently and kept quite short at all times. Unfortunately, though, grass adapts to being cut short, and over time it learns to flower – which is when it produces pollen – closer and closer to the ground. The only answer is to keep a close eye on your lawn and have it cut – and edged, too – as soon as you see signs that it may be starting to flower. You should never mow the lawn yourself if you suffer from hayfever, even if it is not flowering, because doing so releases small allergens that are similar to grass pollen and lead to a cross-reaction (see pages 20-21). Remember to edge the lawn each time as well.

FLOWERS

Garden flowers are rarely the direct cause of hayfever, since they are pollinated by insects rather than the

Tagetes officinalis (marigold) is a member of the daisy family and should be avoided by hayfever sufferers.

wind (see pages 16-17), but they are often capable of causing a cross-reaction (see pages 20-21) if they are from the same botanical family as the plants that produce pollen to which you are allergic. Look in a botanical book to check which plants are close relatives of the ones that cause you problems: in general, if you suffer from hayfever you should avoid planting ornamental grasses, or flowers in the daisy family, such as chrysanthemums, marigolds, asters and sunflowers. And stay clear of goldenrod if you are allergic to ragweed.

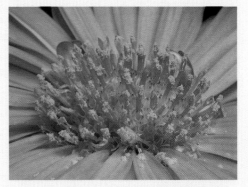

An aster flower in close-up, showing the stamens and pollen. This is another flower to be avoided by allergic gardeners.

TREES

Normally, you have to live with any trees that are in your garden or overhang it, but if you have any choice in the matter avoid birches, alders and hazels. The catkins on hazel and alder trees also affect many of those who have hayfever and so should be avoided – take care, too, that you don't bring them inside the house in the guise of flower decorations. Sometimes hedges that contain cypresses are the cause of hayfever problems, in which case the cypresses should be cut down and replaced with other shrubs, or even a wooden fence.

FURTHER MEASURES

Tidiness is an important consideration in the garden of an allergic person. Make sure there are no untidy areas of wilderness: use weedkiller to keep weeds at bay. Disposing of garden rubbish is also a problem because compost heaps can encourage mould formation (which will cause an allergic reaction in some people) and a bonfire can cover a large area with allergenic particles. Instead, put grass cuttings in bags, seal the bags and take them – or persuade someone who is not sensitive to grass pollen to take them – to the local dump.

The seeds of Helianthus annus (sunflower) can cause a cross-reaction in people who are allergic to ragweed.

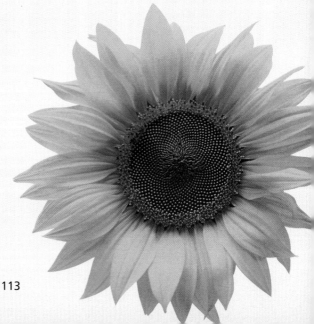

Pollen avoidance

The following tables provide a month-by-month listing of the main sources of pollen for most parts of the world. They will tell you the best time and place for a holiday so that you can avoid the pollen that most affects you.

KEY

G	Grasses	S	Shrubs and
T	Trees and tree crops		hedging plants
W	Weeds	C	Crops

GREAT BRITAIN AND IRELAND

MONTH		PLANT NAME
February-March	T	Ulmus (elm)
February-April	T	Alnus (alder)
	T	Carpinus (hornbeam)
	T	Corylus (hazel)
March-May	T	Populus (poplar)
	T	Salix (willow)
April-May	S	Myrica gale (bog myrtle)
	T	Acer (maple and sycamore)
	T	Aesculus (horse chestnut)
	T	Betula (birches)
	T	Fagus (beech)
	T	Fraxinus (ash)
	T	Pineaceae (pine)
	T	Platanus (plane)
	T	Quercus (oak)
April-September	W	Asteraceae (dandelion)
	W	Compositae (goldenrod)
May-June	T	Juglans (walnut)
	S	Ligustrum (privet)
May-July	S	Sambucus (elder)
	W	Rumex (dock and sorrel)
	G	Gramineae
	G	Poaceae
May-October	W	Amaranthaceae (amaranth)
	W	Chenopodiaceae (goosefoot)
June-July	T	Castanea (chestnut)
June-September	W	Parietaria (pellitory-of-the-wall)
	W	Ambrosia (ragweed)
	W	Urtica (nettle)
July-September	S	Erica, Calluna (heathers)
	C	Oil-seed rape
	W	Artemisia (mugwort, wormwood)

SCANDANAVIA

This area includes Finland, Sweden, Norway and Denmark.

MONTH		PLANT NAME
March-May	T	Ulmus (elms)
April-May	T	Alnus (alder)
	T	Corylus (hazel)
	T	Myrica gale (bog myrtle or sweet gale)
April-June	T	Betula (birches)
May	T	Fraxinus (ash trees)
May-June	T	Quercus (oaks)
May-July	T	Pinaceae (pines)
	T	Cupressaceae (cypresses)
May-August	G	Gramineae
	G	Poaceae
June-August	T	Plantago (plantains)
	W	Rumex (docks)
	W	Urtica (nettles)
July-September	S	Artemisia (mugwort and wormwoods)

NORTHERN AND EASTERN EUROPE

This area includes Austria, Belgium, Czechoslovakia, northern France, Germany, Hungary, Luxembourg, the Netherlands, Poland and Switzerland.

MONTH		PLANT NAME
February-May	T	Alnus (alder)
	T	Carpinus (hornbeam)
	T	Corylus (hazel)
	T	Cupressaceae (cypresses)
March-April	T	Taxus (yew)
March-May	T	Platanus (plane trees)
April-May	T	Betula (birches)
	T	Fraxinus (ash trees)
April-June	T	Fagus (beeches)
	T	Quercus (oaks)
April-July	T	Pinaceae (pines)

April-September	G	Gramineae
	G	Poaceae
May-August	W	Rumex (docks and sorrels)
May-September	W	Pellitories (parietaria)
	T	Plantagago (plantains)
May-October	W	Amaranthaceae (amaranths)
	W	Chenopodiaceae (goosefoots)
June-July	T	Castanea (chestnut trees)
June-September	W	Urtica (nettles)
July-September	S	Artemisia (mugwort and wormwoods)
August-September	W	Ambrosia (ragweeds)

SPAIN & PORTUGAL

MONTH		PLANT NAME
January-March	T	Cupressaceae (cypresses)
February-March	T	Alnus (alder)
February-May	T	Fraxinus (ash trees)
March, April or May	T	Platanus (plane trees)
March-June	T	Plantago (plantains)
	T	Quercus (oaks)
March-July	T	Pinaceae (pines)
March-May or May-July	W	Pellitories (parietaria)
April	T	Betula (birches)
April-June	G	Gramineae Poaceae
May-June	T	Olea (olive trees)
	T	Eucalyptus (eucalyptus or gum trees)
May-July	W	Urtica (nettles)
May-September	W	Amaranthaceae (amaranths)
	W	Chenopodiaceae (goosefoots)
June-August	C	Helianthus (sunflowers)
August-September	S	Artemisia (mugwort and wormwoods)
October-November	T	Casuarina (she-oaks or 'Australian pines')

ACKNOWLEDGEMENTS

In preparing this chart, the publisher would like to acknowledge information published by Dr Jean Emberlin of the Pollen Research Unit at the University of North London, Professor Eugenio Dominguez-Vilches of the University of Cordoba, and Professor Walter H. Lewis and Dr Prathiba Vinay of Washington University.

THE MEDITTERRANEAN

This area covers southern France, Greece, Italy and the Mediterranean islands. (The information supplied for Turkey and the Balkans may be more applicable for northeastern Greece.)

MONTH		PLANT NAME
January-May	T	Alnus (alder)
	T	Corylus (hazel)
February-May	T	Acacia (mimosa)
March-April	T	Populus (poplars)
March-July	T	Olea (olive trees)
	T	Pinaceae (pines)
	W	Parietaria (pellitories)
April-May	T	Betula (birches)
	T	Broussonetia papyrifera (paper mulberry)
April-June	T	Quercus (oaks)
	W	Urtica (nettles)
April-September	G	Gramineae Poaceae
	W	Rumex (docks and sorrel)
May-September	T	Plantago (plantains)
May-October	W	Amaranthaceae (amaranths)
	W	Chenopodiaceae (goosefoots)
June-July	T	Castanea (chestnuts)
August-September	W	Ambrosia (ragweeds)
August-October	S	Artemisia (mugwort and wormwoods)
September-November	W	Parietaria (pellitories)
December-June	T	Cupressaceae (cypresses)

THE CANARY ISLANDS

MONTH		PLANT NAME
April	G	Grasses

TURKEY AND THE BALKANS

This area includes Bulgaria, Romania, Turkey and the countries of the former Yugoslavia.

MONTH		PLANT NAME
February-May	T	Alnus (alder)
	T	Carpinus (hornbeam)
	T	Corylus (hazel)
	T	Ostrya (hop-hornbeam)
March-April	T	Populus (poplars)
	T	Fraxinus (ash trees)

March-May	T	*Acer negundo* (box elder or ash-leaved maple)
	T	*Cupressaceae* (cypresses)
March-August	W	*Urtica* (nettles)
April-May	T	*Betula* (birches)
	T	*Fagus* (beeches)
	T	*Platanus* (plane trees)
April-May	T	*Quercus* (oaks)
	T	*Erica arborea* (tree heather)
April-June	W	*Rumex* (docks and sorrels)
April-July	T	*Pinaceae* (pines)
May-June	T	*Olea* (olive trees)
May-August	T	*Plantago* (plantains)
	W	*Pellitories* (parietaria)
May-September	G	*Gramineae*
	G	*Poaceae*
June-October	W	*Amaranthaceae* (amaranths)
	W	*Chenopodiaceae* (goosefoots)
July-September	S	*Artemisia* (mugwort and wormwoods)
August-September	W	*Ambrosia* (ragweeds)
September-October	T	*Erica arborea* (tree heather)

THE FORMER USSR

In Russia (west of the Urals), Bielarus, the Ukraine and the Caucasus region, the pollen seasons are similar to eastern Europe (see pages 114-115). No information regarding the other countries in this region.

THE MIDDLE EAST

Lebanon, and western Jordan and Syria.

MONTH		PLANT NAME
March-May	G	Grasses
May-June	T	*Olea* (olive trees)
August-October	S	*Artemisia* (mugwort)

ISRAEL

MONTH		PLANT NAME
March-June	G	Grasses
May-June	T	*Olea* (olive trees)

IRAN

MONTH		PLANT NAME
November-February	T	*Cupressaceae* (cypresses)

EGYPT (ALEXANDRIA REGION)

MONTH		PLANT NAME
mid-February-early December	G	Grasses
late February-November	W	*Chenopodiaceae* (goosefoot)
	W	*Urtica* (nettles)

INDIA & PAKISTAN

Except for the far south, February-April will have the lowest pollen counts. Some level of pollen throughout the remaining months.

NORTH AFRICA

The northern coast of Morocco, Algeria and Tunisia.

MONTH		PLANT NAME
March-May	G	Grasses
May	T	*Olea* (olive trees)

WEST AFRICA

The savanna region from the rainforests north to the Sahel, Nigeria and northern Ghana.

MONTH		PLANT NAME
April-November	G	Grasses

EAST AFRICA – KENYA

MONTH		PLANT NAME
September-October,	G	Grasses
December-January	G	Grasses

EAST AFRICA – THE SAVANNAS OF TANZANIA

MONTH		PLANT NAME
June-December	G	Grasses

EAST AFRICA – ZIMBABWEE

MONTH		PLANT NAME
all year round but peaking in July-August, October-November	G	Grasses

EAST AFRICA – MALAWI

MONTH		PLANT NAME
October-February	G	Grasses

SOUTHERN AFRICA – BOTSWANA

MONTH		PLANT NAME
November-April	G	Grasses

SOUTH AFRICA

Most months of the year peaking:

SOUTH AFRICA – CAPE TOWN

MONTH		PLANT NAME
November-January	G	Grasses

SOUTH AFRICA – JOHANNESBURG AND PRETORIA

MONTH		PLANT NAME
December-January	G	Grasses

JAPAN

MONTH		PLANT NAME
February-April	T	*Cryptomeria japonica* (Japanese red cedar)
February-May	T	*Betula* (birches)
March-April	T	*Alnus* (alders)
	T	*Cupressaceae* (cypresses)
April-June	G	*Gramineae*
	G	*Poaceae*
July-August	W	*Ambrosia* (ragweed)
	C	*Humulus* (hops)
July-September	S	*Artemisia* (mugwort)
August-September	T	*Plantago* (plantains)
	W	*Chenopodiaceae* (goosefoot)
	W	*Urtica* (nettles)

AUSTRALIA – WESTERN AUSTRALIA

MONTH		PLANT NAME
May-February	T	*Acacia* (wattles)
July-November	T	*Casuarina* (she-oak or 'Australian pine')
	T	*Pinaceae* (pines)
	W	*Arctotheca calendula* (capeweed)
August-February	T	*Plantago* (plantains)
August-October	T	*Callitris columellaris* (white cypress pine)
	T	*Cupressaceae* (cypresses)
August-November	S	*Ligustrum* (privet)
September-January	W	*Rumex* (docks and sorrels)
September-February	W	*Chenopodiaceae* (goosefoots)

September-March	G	*Gramineae*
	G	*Poaceae*
October-February	C	*Helianthus* (sunflower)
October-March	T	*Eucalyptus* (gum trees)
October-November	W	*Echium plantagineum* (Peterson's curse or Salvation Jane)
November-December	T	*Olea* (olive trees)

AUSTRALIA – NORTHERN TERRITORY

MONTH		PLANT NAME
October-March	G	*Gramineae*
	G	*Poaceae*

AUSTRALIA – QUEENSLAND

MONTH		PLANT NAME
January-December	T	*Eucalyptus* (gum trees)
May-October	T	*Acacia* (wattles)
August-March	T	*Plantago* (plantains)
September-February	T	*Casuarina* (she-oak or 'Australian pine')
	W	*Rumex* (docks and sorrels)
September-April	W	*Chenopodiaceae* (goosefoots)
September-May	G	*Gramineae*
	G	*Poaceae*
September-November	S	*Ligustrum* (privet)
	T	*Callitris columellaris* (white cypress pine or Murray pine)
October-November	W	*Arctotheca calendula* (capeweed)
December-May	C	*Helianthus* (sunflower)

AUSTRALIA – NEW SOUTH WALES

MONTH		PLANT NAME
January-December	T	*Eucalyptus* (gum trees)
June-February	T	*Plantago* (plantains)
June-April	W	*Parietaria judaica* (pellitory-of-the-wall)
June-December	T	*Acacia* (wattles)
July-April	T	*Casuarina* (she-oak or 'Australian pine')
August-May	G	*Gramineae*
	G	*Poaceae*
August-November	T	*Callitris columellaris* (white cypress pine or Murray pine)

August-November	T	Cupressaceae (cypresses)
September-February	W	Rumex (docks and sorrels)
September-October	T	Betula pendula (silver birch)
September-November	S	Ligustrum (privet)
	W	Arctotheca calendula (capeweed)
September-December	W	Echium plantagineum (Paterson's curse or Salvation Jane)
October-November	T	Olea (olive trees)
December-January	W	Artemisia (wormwood)
December-February	W	Chenopodiaceae (goosefoots)
December-May	C	Helianthus (sunflower)

AUSTRALIA – VICTORIA

MONTH		PLANT NAME
January-December	T	Eucalyptus (gum trees)
March-April	T	Casuarina (she-oak or 'Australian pine')
April-September	T	Cupressaceae (cypresses)
June-October	T	Callitris columellaris (white cypress pine or Murray pine)
July-January	T	Acacia (wattles)
July-August	T	Casuarina
August-February	W	Rumex (docks and sorrels)
August-September	T	Pinaceae (pines)
August-December	W	Arctotheca calendula (capeweed)
	W	Echium plantagineum (Paterson's curse or Salvation Jane)
September-February	W	Trifolium (clover)
September-May	G	Gramineae
	G	Poaceae
September-October	T	Betula pendula (silver birch)
October-March	T	Plantago (plantains)
October-November	T	Olea (olive trees)
October-December	S	Ligustrum (privet)
December-April	W	Chenopodiaceae (goosefoots)

AUSTRALIA – SOUTH AUSTRALIA

MONTH		PLANT NAME
March-July	T	Casuarina (she-oak or 'Australian pine')
July-March	G	Gramineae
July-March	G	Poaceae
July-November	T	Acacia (wattles)
July-December	W	Echium plantagineum (Paterson's curse or Salvation Jane)
August-March	T	Eucalyptus (gum trees)
	T	Plantago (plantains)
August-September	T	Casuarina (she-oak or 'Australian pine')
August-October	T	Callitris columellaris (white cypress pine or Murray pine)
	T	Cupressaceae (cypresses)
August-November	W	Arctotheca calendula (capeweed)
September-February	W	Trifolium (clover)
September-November	T	Betula pendula (silver birch)
	T	Olea (olive trees)
	S	Ligustrum (privet)
September-December	W	Rumex (docks and sorrels)
December-April	W	Chenopodiaceae (goosefoots)

AUSTRALIA – TASMANIA

MONTH		PLANT NAME
June-December	T	Casuarina (she-oak or 'Australian pine')
July-November	T	Cupressaceae (cypresses)
	T	Pinaceae (pines)
August-February	T	Acacia (wattles)
	T	Eucalyptus (gum trees)
September-January	W	Arctotheca calendula (capeweed)
September-April	G	Gramineae
	G	Poaceae
September-May	W	Rumex (docks and sorrels)
September-November	T	Betula pendula (silver birch)
October-March	T	Plantago (plantains)

NEW ZEALAND

MONTH		PLANT NAME
January-March	W	Rumex (docks and sorrels)
July-October	T	Pinaceae (pines)
July-November	T	Cupressaceae (cypresses)
August-October	T	Betula (birches)
	T	Quercus (oaks)
August-November	T	Acacia (wattles)
August-November	T	Albizia (mimosas)
October-February	G	Gramineae
	G	Poaceae
		Plantago (plantains)
October-March	S	Ligustrum (privet)

HAWAII

MONTH		PLANT NAME
January-December (except late December)	G	Gramineae
	G	Poaceae
January-April	T	Various native and introduced species especially:
	T	Cryptomeria (Japanese red cedar)
	T	Eucalyptus (gum trees)
May (mid)-December	W	Weeds

CANADA – ALASKA (USA) AND NORTH CANADA

MONTH		PLANT NAME
April-May	T	Alnus (alder)
	T	Populus (poplars)
	T	Salix (willows)
April-June	T	Myrica gale (bog myrtle or sweet gale)
May-June	T	Betula (birches)
May-September	G	Gramineae
	G	Poaceae

CANADA – NORTHEAST

This area covers northern Ontario, northern Quebec, Labrador and Newfoundland.

MONTH		PLANT NAME
April-June	T	Myrica gale (bog myrtle or sweet gale)
May-June	T	Betula (birches)
July	G	Gramineae
	G	Poaceae
July-August	T	Pinaceae (spruce, fir and larch)

CANADA – SOUTHEAST

This area covers southern Ontario, southern Quebec, New Brunswick and Nova Scotia.

MONTH		PLANT NAME
April	T	Alnus (alders)
April-May	T	Fraxinus (ash trees)
	T	Populus (poplars)
	T	Salix (willows)
April-June	T	Morus (mulberry)
	T	Myrica gale (bog myrtle or sweet gale)
May-June	T	Acer (maples)
	T	Betula (birches)
	T	Carya (hickories)
	T	Celtis (hackberries)
	T	Fagus (beeches)
	T	Quercus (oaks)
	T	Ulmus (elms)
	S	Ligustrum (privet)
May-August	G	Gramineae
	G	Poaceae
June-August	T	Pinaceae (pines and spruces)
July	T	Tilia (lindens and basswoods)
July-September	W	Chenopodiaceae (goosefoots, pigweed and 'Russian thistle')
July-October	T	Plantago (plantains)
August-September	W	Ambrosia (ragweeds)
	W	Artemisia (mugwort and wormwoods)

BRITISH COLUMBIA

MONTH		PLANT NAME
February-June	T	Cupressaceae (cypresses, junipers and 'cedars'
April-May	T	Alnus (alders)
	T	Populus (poplars)
	T	Salix (willows)
April-June	T	Myrica gale (bog myrtle or sweet gale)
May-June	T	Acer (maples)
	T	Betula (birches)
May-September	G	Gramineae
	G	Poaceae
August-September	W	Ambrosia (ragweeds)

GREAT PLAINS OF CANADA

This area covers Alberta, Saskatchewan and Manitoba.

MONTH		PLANT NAME
March-June	T	Cupressaceae (cypresses, junipers and 'cedars'
April-May	T	Betula (birches)
	T	Populus (poplars and quaking aspen)
April-June	T	Myrica gale (bog myrtle or sweet gale)
May	T	Quercus (oaks)
May-June	T	Acer (maples)
	T	Ulmus (elms)
May-August	G	Gramineae
	G	Poaceae
August-September	T	Plantago (plantains)
	W	Ambrosia (ragweeds)
	W	Artemisia (mugwort and wormwoods)
	W	Chenopodiaceae (goosefoots)

USA – WASHINGTON AND OREGON

MONTH		PLANT NAME
February-April	T	Alnus (alder)
March-May	T	Cupressaceae (cypresses, junipers and 'cedars')
	T	Populus (poplars)
	T	Salix (willows)
	T	Sequoia (coast redwood)
April-May	T	Acer (maples)
	T	Betula (birches)
	T	Quercus (oaks)
April-September	G	Gramineae
	G	Poaceae
May-September	W	Rumex (docks and sorrels)
May-November	T	Plantago (plantains)
June-October	W	Amaranthaceae (amaranths)
	W	Chenopodiaceae (goosefoots)
July-October	W	Ambrosia (ragweeds)

USA – CALIFORNIA

MONTH		PLANT NAME
January-September	W	Urtica (nettles)
January-October	T	Acacia (wattles and acacias)
January-December	W	Rumex (docks and sorrels)

February-April	T	Fraxinus (ash)
	T	Quercus (oaks)
	T	Ulmus (elms)
February-May	T	Myrica (Bayberry or wax myrtle)
	T	Casuarina (she-oak or 'Australian pine')
February-July	W	Parietaria (pellitories)
March-April	T	Cryptomeria (Japanese red cedar)
March-May	T	Acer (maples)
	T	Broussonetia (paper mulberry)
	T	Carya (hickories)
	T	Juglans (walnuts and pecans)
	T	Morus (mulberry)
March-June	S	Ligustrum (privet)
April-May	T	Populus (poplars)
April-October	G	Gramineae
	G	Poaceae
April-December	W	Amaranthaceae (amaranths)
	W	Ambrosia (ragweeds)
	W	Chenopodiaceae (goosefoots)
May-June	T	Olea (olive trees)
May-July	S	Prosopis (mesquite)
May-November	T	Plantago (plantains)
June-December	T	Arecaceae (palm trees)
July-September	W	Artemisia (sagebrush)
August-October	T	Ulmus (elms)
August-November	W	Iva (poverty weeds and marsh elders)
September-March	T	Cupressaceae (cypresses, junipers and 'cedars')
September-November	T	Casuarina (she-oak or 'Australian pine')
December-March	T	Eucalyptus (gum trees)
December-May	T	Alnus (alders)
	T	Betula (birches)

USA – MONTANA, IDAHO AND WYOMING

MONTH		PLANT NAME
January-February	T	Cupressaceae (cypresses)
February-April	T	Alnus (alders)
	T	Carpinus (hornbeams)
	T	Corylus (hazels)
	T	Ostrya (ironwood)
March-May	T	Populus (poplars)
	T	Salix (willows)
April-May	T	Betula (birches)

April-May	T	Quercus (oaks)
May-September	G	Gramineae
	G	Poaceae
May-November	T	Plantago (plantains)
	W	Rumex (docks and sorrels)
June-October	W	Amaranthaceae (amaranths)
	W	Chenopodiaceae (goosefoots)
August-September	W	Ambrosia (ragweeds)
	W	Artemisia (sagebrush)

USA – NEVADA, UTAH AND COLORADO

MONTH		PLANT NAME
January-March	T	Cupressaceae (cypresses, junipers and 'cedars'
March-October	G	Gramineae
	G	Poaceae
April-May	T	Populus (poplars)
May-September	W	Rumex (docks and sorrels)
June-October	W	Amaranthaceae (amaranths)
	W	Chenopodiaceae (goosefoots)
July-September	W	Parietaria (pellitories)
August-September	W	Ambrosia (ragweeds)

USA – ARIZONA AND NEW MEXICO

MONTH		PLANT NAME
February-March	T	Fraxinus (ash trees)
February-November	G	Gramineae
	G	Poaceae
March-September	W	Rumex (docks and sorrels)
April-October	W	Amaranthaceae (amaranths)
	W	Chenopodiaceae (goosefoots)
May-June	T	Olea (olive trees)
May-July	S	Prosopia (mesquite)
July-September	W	Artemisia (sagebrush)
August-September	W	Ambrosia (ragweeds)
	W	Franseria (bur ragweed)
September-March	T	Cupressaceae (cypresses, junipers and 'cedars')

USA – THE SOUTH

This area includes Texas, Louisiana, Mississippi and Alabama.

MONTH		PLANT NAME
January-April	T	Celtis (hackberries and sugarberries)
	T	Ulmus (elms)
February-May	T	Acer (maples)
March-April	T	Myrica cerifera (Southern bayberry or wax myrtle)
March-May	T	Broussonetica (paper mulberry)
	T	Carya (hickories and pecans)
	T	Morus (mulberries)
March-June	S	Ligustrum (privet)
March-December	G	Gramineae
	G	Poaceae
April-June	S	Maclura (hedgeplant or osage orange)
June-December	W	Amaranthaceae (amaranths)
	W	Chenopodiaceae (goosefoots)
July-November	W	Ambrosia (ragweeds)
August-October	T	Celtis (hackberries and sugarberries)
	T	Ulmus (elms)
August-November	T	Baccharis halmilifolia (groundsel bush or tree)
	W	Iva (marsh elders and dune elder)
September-March	T	Cupressaceae (junipers and 'cedars')

USA – SOUTH-CENTRAL STATES

This area includes Kansas , Oklahoma, Missouri and Arkansas.

MONTH		PLANT NAME
February-March	T	Celtis (hackberries and sugarberries)
		Fraxinus (ash)
February-May	T	Acer (maples)
March-April	T	Myrica cerifera (southern bayberry or wax myrtle)
March-May	T	Betula (birches)
	T	Broussonetia papyrifera (paper mulberry)
April-May	T	Quercus (oaks)
	S	Maclura (osage orange or hedgeplant)

April-October	W	Amaranthaceae (amaranths)
	W	Chenopodiaceae (goosefoots)
April-November	G	Gramineae
	G	Poaceae
May-September	W	Rumex (docks and sorrels)
May-November	T	Plantago (plantains)
July-September	W	Artemisia (sagebrush)
August-September	W	Ambrosia (ragweeds)

USA – KENTUCKY AND TENNESSEE

MONTH		PLANT NAME
January-March	T	Cupressaceae ('cedars' and junipers)
February-March	T	Acer (maples)
March-April	T	Salix (willows)
April-May	T	Quercus (oaks)
April-September	W	Rumex (docks and sorrels)
May-August	G	Gramineae
	G	Poaceae
May-November	T	Plantago (plantains)
August-October	W	Ambrosia (ragweeds)
	W	Artemisia (wormwoods)

USA – THE MID-WEST

This area includes North and South Dakota, Nebraska, Minnesota, Michigan, Wisconsin, Iowa, Indiana and Idaho.

MONTH		PLANT NAME
February-April	T	Alnus (alder)
	T	Carpinus (ironwood)
	T	Corylus (hazel)
	T	Ostrya (hornbeam)
March-April	T	Populus (poplars)
	T	Salix (willows)
	T	Ulmus (elms)
April-May	T	Acer (maples)
	T	Betula (birches)
	T	Fraxinus (ash trees)
	T	Quercus (oaks)
May-June	S	Ligustrum (privet)
May-July	G	Gramineae
	G	Poaceae
May-September	W	Rumex (docks and sorrels)
May-November	T	Plantago (plantains)
June-September	W	Cannabis sativa (hemp or cannabis)
June-October	W	Amaranthaceae (amaranths)

June-October	W	Chenopodiaceae (goosefoots)
July-September	W	Parietaria (pellitories)
	W	Pilea (clearweed)
	W	Urtica (nettles)
July-October	W	Ambrosia (ragweeds)

USA – THE NORTH EAST AND NEW ENGLAND

This area covers Maine, New Hampshire, Vermont, Massachusetts, Connecticut, Rhode Island, Pennsylvania, New York State, New Jersey, Delaware and Virginia.

MONTH		PLANT NAME
February-April	T	Ulmus (elms)
February-May	T	Acer (maples)
March-April	T	Populus (poplars)
	T	Salix (willows)
March-May	T	Cupressaceae ('cedars' and junipers)
April-May	T	Alnus (alder)
	T	Betula (birches)
	T	Carpinus (ironwood)
	T	Corylus (hazels)
	T	Ostrya (hornbeams)
	T	Pinaceae (pines)
	T	Quercus (oaks and beeches)
April-June	S	Comptonia peregrina (sweet fern)
April-July	T	Myrica (bayberry or wax myrtle)
May	T	Fraxinus (ash trees)
May-June	S	Ligustrum (privet)
May-July	G	Gramineae
	G	Poaceae
May-September	W	Rumex (docks and sorrels)
May-October	W	Pilea (clearwood)
	W	Urtica (nettles)
June-July	T	Tilia (lindens or basswoods)
June-August	T	Plantago (plantains)
June-October	W	Amaranthaceae (amaranths)
	W	Chenopodiaceae (goosefoots)
	W	Parietaria (pellitories)
July-October	W	Ambrosia (ragweeds)
August-October	W	Iva (marsh elders)

USA – THE SOUTHEAST STATES

This area includes North Carolina, South Carolina, Georgia and Florida.

MONTH		PLANT NAME
January-June	W	Parietaria (pellitories)
February-April	T	Betula (birches)
	T	Casuarina (she-oaks or 'Australian pines'
February-May	T	Quercus (oaks)
March-May	T	Acer (maples)
	T	Populus (poplars)
	T	Salix (willows)
	T	Ulmus (elms)
March-June	T	Broussonetia papyrifera (paper mulberry)
March-October	G	Gramineae
	G	Poaceae
April-May	T	Carya (hickories)
	T	Juglans (walnuts)
	S	Maclura (osaga orange or hedgeplant)
April-June	T	Acoelorrhaphe wrightii (everglades palm)
	T	Albizia (mimosa or silk tree)
	W	Rumex (docks and sorrels)
April-October	W	Amaranthaceae (amaranths)
	W	Chenopodiaceae (goosefoots)
May-June	S	Ligustrum (privet)
May-November	T	Plantago (plantains)
July-November	W	Ambrosia (ragweeds)
August-September	W	Iva (marsh elders and dune elder)
August-October	W	Pilea (clearweed)
	W	Urtica (nettles)
October-December	T	Casuarina (she-oaks or 'Australian pines'
	T	Myrica (bayberry or wax myrtle)
December-March	T	Cupressaceae ('cedars', cypresses and junipers)
	T	Eucalyptus (gum trees)
	T	Taxodium (bald 'cypress', or swamp 'cypress' and pond 'cypress')
December-June	T	Pinaceae (pines)

CARIBBEAN

MONTH		PLANT NAME
February-April	T	Casuarina (she-oaks or 'Australian pines')
March-June	W	Urtica (nettles)
April-May	T	Broussonetia papyrifera (paper mulberry)
June-July	G	Gramineae
	G	Poaceae
June-October	T	Celtis (sugarberry or hackberry trees)
October-March	G	Gramineae
	G	Poaceae
December-August	W	Parietaria judaica (pellitory-of-the-wall)

SOUTH AMERICA

In countries north of the equator, such as Venezuela.

MONTH		PLANT NAME
April-July	G	Grasses

NORTHERN BRAZIL

MONTH		PLANT NAME
October-December	G	Grasses

RIO DE JANEIRO

MONTH		PLANT NAME
December-March	G	Grasses

ECUADOR

MONTH		PLANT NAME
January-December	G	Grasses

PERU

MONTH		PLANT NAME
October-January	G	Grasses

ARGENTINA

MONTH		PLANT NAME
October-February	G	Grasses

Useful addresses

The following addresses will offer practical help and advice on finding a natural health practioner, and the stockists and manufacturers of equipment that help relieve the symptoms of hayfever.

ACUPUNCTURE

United Kingdom
British Acupuncture
Council
Park House
206-208 Latimer Road
London W10 6RE
Tel: (44) 0181 964 0222

North America
American Association for
Acupuncture
4101 Lake Boone Trail
Suite 201
Raleigh
North Carolina 27607
USA
Tel: (001) 919 787 5181

Australasia
New Zealand Register of
Acupuncturists
PO Box 9950
Wellington 1
New Zealand
Tel: 64 4 476 8578

ALEXANDER TECHNIQUE

United Kingdom
Society of Teachers of the
Alexander Technique
20 London House
266 Fulham Road
London SW10 9EL
Tel:(44) 0171 351 0828

North America
North American Society of
Teachers of the Alexander
Technique
PO Box 517
Urbana
Illinois 61801-0517
USA
Tel: (001) 217 367 6956

Canada
Canadian Society of
Teachers of the Alexander
Technique
PO Box 47025
19-555 West 12th Avenue
Vancouver
British Columbia V5Z 3 XO
Canada

Australasia
Australian Society of
Teachers of the Alexander
Technique
PO Box 716
Darlinghurst
New South Wales 2010
Australia
Tel: 61 8339 571

AROMATHERAPY

United Kingdom
International Federation
of Aromatherapists
Stamford House
2-4 Chiswick High Road
London W4 1TH
Tel: (44) 0181 742 2605

North America
American Aromatherapy
Association
PO Box 3679
South Pasadena
California 91031
USA
Tel: (001) 818 457 1742

BACH FLOWER REMEDIES

United Kingdom
Dr Edward Bach Centre
Mount Vernon
Sotwell
Wallingford
Oxon OX10 0PZ
Great Britain
Tel: (44) 01491 834678

North America
Dr Edward Bach Healing
Society
644 Merrick Road
Lynbrook
New York
USA
Tel: (001) 516 593 2206

Australasia
Martin & Pleasance
137 Swan Street
Richmond
Victoria 3121
Australia
Tel: 61 39 427 7422

HERBALISM
United Kingdom
School of Herbal Medicine
Bucksteep Manor
Bodle Street Green
Near Hailsham
Sussex BN27 4RJ
Great Britain
Tel: (44) 01323 834 800

North America
American Herbalists Guild
PO Box 1683
Soquel
California 95073
USA

Australasia
National Herbalists
Association of Australia
Suite 305
BST House
3 Smail Street
Broadway
New South Wales 2007
Australia
Tel: 61 2 211 6437

HOMEOPATHY
United Kingdom
British Homeopathic
Association
27A Devonshire Street
London W1N 1RJ
Great Britain
Tel: (44) 0171 935 2163

North America
National Center for
Homeopathy
801 N Fairfax Street
Alexandria
VA 22314
USA
Tel: (001) 703 548 7790

HYDROTHERAPY
United Kingdom
UK College of
Hydrotherapy
515 Hagley Road
Birmingham B66 4AX
Great Britain
Tel: (44) 0121 429 9191

North America
Aquatic Exercise
Association
PO Box 1609
Nokomis
Florida 34274
USA
Tel: (001) 813 486 8600

HYPNOTHERAPY
United Kingdom
British Hypnotherapy
Association
67 Upper Berkeley Street
London
W1H 7DH
Great Britain
Tel: (44) 0171 723 4443

North America
American Association of
Professional
Hypnotherapists
PO Box 29
Boones Mill
Virginia 24065
USA
Tel: (001) 703 334 3035

MASSAGE
United Kingdom
British Massage Therapy
Council
Greenbank House
65a Adelphi Street
Preston PR1 7BH
Great Britain
Tel: (44) 01772 881 063

North America
National Association of
Massage Therapy
PO Box 1400
Westminster
Colorado 80030-1400
USA
Tel: (001) 800 776 6268

Australasia
Association of Massage
Therapists
18a Spit Road
Mosman
New South Wales
Australia
Tel: 02 969 8445

NATUROPATHY
United Kingdom
General Council and
Register of Naturopaths
Goswell House
2 Goswell Road
Street
Somerset BA16 0JG
Great Britain
Tel: (44) 01458 840072

North America
American Association of
Naturopathic Physicians
PO Box 20386
Seattle
Washington 98102
USA
Tel: (001) 205 323 7610

Canadian Naturopathic
Association
205, 1234 17th Avenue
South West
PO Box 4143
Station C
Calgary
Alberta
Canada
Tel: (001) 413 244 4487

Australasia
Australian Natural
Therapists Association
PO Box 522
Sutherland
New South Wales
Australia
Tel: 02 521 2063

New Zealand Natural
Health Practitioners
Accreditation Board
PO Box 37-491
Auckland
New Zealand
Te: 64 9 625 9966

REFLEXOLOGY

United Kingdom
Association of
Reflexologists
27 Old Gloucester Street
London WC1N 3XX
Great Britain
Tel: (44) 0990 673 320

North America
International Institute of
Reflexology
PO Box 12642
Saint Petersberg
Florida 33733
USA
Tel: (001) 813 343 4811

Reflexology Association of
Canada
11 Glen Cameron Road
Unit 4
Thornhill
Ontario L8T 4NE
Canada
Tel: (001) 905 889 5900

Australasia
Reflexology Association of
Australia
15 Kedumba Crescent
Turramurra 2074
New South Wales
Australia

New Zealand Reflexology
Association
PO Box 31 084
Auckland 4
New Zealand

POLLEN FORECASTS

United Kingdom
Pollen Research Unit
University of North
London
166-220 Holloway Rd
London N8 8DB
Great Britain
Tel: (44) 0171 607 2789

Australasia
Pollen Monitoring Dept
University of Otago
Dunedin
New Zealand

SELF-HELP GROUPS

United Kingdom
The British Allergy
Foundation
Deepdene House
30 Bellegrove Rd
Welling
Kent DA16 3PY
Great Britain
Tel: (44) 0181 303 8525

Australasia
Allergy Association,
Australia
PO Box 298
Ringwood
Victoria 314
Australia

Allergy Awareness
Association
PO Box 120701
Penrose
Auckland 6
New Zealand

STOCKISTS & MANUFACTURERS

United Kingdom
Dyson Appliances
Tetbury Hill
Malmesbury
Wilts SN16 0RP
Great Britain
Tel: (44) 01666 827 272

Medivac plc
Wilmslow House
Grove Way
Wilmslow
Cheshire SK9 5AG
Great Britain
Tel: (44) 01625 539 401

The Healthy House
Cold Harbour
Ruscombe
Stroud
Glos GL6 6DA
Great Britain
Tel: (44) 01453 752 216

Australasia
Protector Safety Pty Ltd
17 Main Road
Wivenhoe
Burnie
Tasmania 7320
Australia

Index

Index compiled by Hilary Bird.